Dr Mike Smith's Handbook of Prescription Medicines

DR MIKE SMITH, a specialist in preventive medicine and President of the Association of Broadcasting Doctors. He was the Chief Medical Officer of the Family Planning Association 1970–75 and their Honorary Medical Adviser 1975–90. He is an elected member of the FPA's National Executive Committee and a member of the advisory panel of both the national Food Safety Advisory Centre and the British Association of Continence Care. For many years he has been a resident expert guest on BBC2's *Jimmy Young Programme*, LBC's *Nightline* and the medical columnist/editor for *Woman's Own*. Between 1980 and 1984 he presented BBC1's health series *Looking Good, Feeling Fit* and from 1988–90 he was the expert guest on SKY TV's *Sky by Day*. In April 1991 he was voted the TV and Radio Doctors' 'Experts' Expert' in the *Observer* magazine's series.

His other books include *Birth Control, How to Save Your Child's Life, A New Dictionary of Symptoms* and the *Dr Mike Smith's Postbag* series. This book is a companion to *Dr Mike Smith's Handbook of Over-the-Counter Medicines* (Kyle Cathie 1992).

By the same author from Kyle Cathie Limited:

DR MIKE SMITH'S POSTBAG:
STRESS
ARTHRITIS
HRT
BACK PAIN

DR MIKE SMITH'S HANDBOOK OF
OVER-THE-COUNTER MEDICINES

Dr Mike Smith's Handbook of Prescription Medicines

Researcher: Sharron Kerr

KYLE CATHIE LIMITED

First published in Great Britain in 1993 by
Kyle Cathie Limited
7/8 Hatherley Street London SW1P 2QT

ISBN 1 85626 105 0

A CIP catalogue record for this book is available from the British Library.

Designed by Beverley Waldron
Typeset by DP Photosetting, Aylesbury, Bucks
Printed in England by Clays Ltd, St Ives plc

Contents

Acknowledgements

For her extensive research on this book, a thousand thanks go to journalist Sharron Kerr, my colleague and friend.

My thanks also go to Joan Tillott MRPhS and Nazleen Meghji MRPharmS of Tillott and Tongue District Pharmacy – my local chemists – and to the pharmaceutical companies who readily sent details of their products.

Introduction

This book is not intended as a medical dictionary, nor as a means for people to diagnose their own illnesses. But what the book does aim to do is help a patient understand what's wrong with them, how they can take steps to prevent the condition occurring again, where possible, what types of medicine are available and what they do (because of the numbers involved it would be impossible to list every one in a book of this nature and size). It's not a substitute for a consultation with your doctor or your pharmacist but more of a complement to a consultation, particularly if there are questions you forgot or were too embarrassed to ask!

And it seems there is a need for more explanation and education about prescription medicines. One survey carried out in the late '80s revealed that more than half of patients questioned didn't know exactly how, when or with what they should take their medicines and about eight in 10 hadn't been warned about potential side-effects. Most patients did state that they wanted to know more about their drugs. Another survey showed that more than half of the patients had been prescribed medicines without their possible side-effects being explained to them.

Fortunately, the situation looks set to change. As a result of a European Community directive there are plans to give people more information on how individual medicines work and how to use them safely and most effectively, by including information leaflets with the packaging. These leaflets are going to be phased in during the next five years or so.

Other changes being developed include the number of medicines GPs are allowed to prescribe under the National Health Service. In 1985 a cost-saving list was introduced restricting GPs' prescribing choice of medicines within certain categories. They are antacids, laxatives, analgesics for mild to moderate pain relief, vitamins and tonics, benzodiazepine sedatives and tranquillisers. However patients must rest assured that they will receive the medication they need as in each category a drug is only blacklisted if there is an equally effective but cheaper equivalent. At the end of last year it was announced that the government intended to extend the Selected List Scheme to include ten new categories of drugs. These include topical anti-rheumatics, anti-diarrhoeal drugs and appetite suppressants, drugs for vaginal and vulval conditions, hypnotics and anxiolytics, drugs acting on the skin, drugs for allergic disorders, drugs used in anaemia, drugs acting on the ear and nose, contraceptives. These categories are currently under discussion.

There is great concern from many interested parties about the proposed changes, within the successful UK pharmaceutical industry (which employs around 90,000 people) in particular, because drug costs are a constant proportion (one tenth) of total NHS spending – less than domestic/cleaning services or catering. And UK spending on drugs is said to be lower than that of other comparable nations. NHS patients average eight prescription items per year compared with 12 in Germany, 20 in Italy and 38 in France.

GPs are concerned that they may only be allowed to prescribe the relatively cheaper, established medicines and consequently newer ones, which may have fewer side-effects, could be blacklisted. Not only that, what may suit one patient may not suit another. Drug efficiency and tolerance vary enormously from patient to patient. Sometimes different medicines need to be prescribed before the most effective individual treatment is reached. Patients are concerned that they might not be able to afford to buy any blacklisted products that they have come to rely on. Support groups are concerned that patients suffering from one type of condition, say eczema, dealt with in the proposed new categories, face discrimination because of this.

Another change that's been developing as part of the new, cost-conscious NHS, is the increase in generically prescribed medicines. If you've been receiving prescriptions for medicines fairly frequently over the last few years, you may have already noticed that the 25,000 GPs in the UK are often prescribing the generic forms of drugs rather than by brand names. Nearly half of all prescriptions currently written are generic and that proportion is steadily rising. With the NHS reforms and the introduction of fund-holding practices, GPs are having to become price conscious when it comes to prescribing. A generic is supposedly the non-branded equivalent of a proprietary, branded drug. Invariably, it's low cost, as generic suppliers only bear the direct cost of manufacture, without the risks of new product development or the costs of gaining the drug's acceptance by doctors – another cause for concern in the pharmaceutical industry.

Taking your medicine Despite all the changes and consequent concerns, when it comes to taking your prescription medicine the advice remains constant. Common sense should prevail at all times. When your doctor hands you a prescription with your name at the top, he or she means it to be taken by you alone – and no one else. It's designed to deal with your problem, not any symptoms of your husband, wife, neighbour or friend. So don't dish out medicines, and don't accept any from anyone else either, no matter how well meaning the person is.

Always remind your doctor if you already have a medical condition when you are being prescribed a medicine, for example, if you have asthma, diabetes, any allergies (to penicillin, for instance, or aspirin intolerance), heart disease, high blood pressure and so on.

If you are pregnant, even if you only think you might be, always tell your doctor. Some medicines may be harmful, particularly if taken during the first 12 weeks of pregnancy, and often there is just not enough evidence that they are safe in pregnancy. Your doctor will then assess your need for a certain medicine. He or she may have to weigh up the benefits of use during pregnancy against the possible hazards to mother and foetus. The same care should also be taken if you are a breast-feeding mother, because some drugs can appear in breast milk.

Some medicines may react with each other, altering their effect so, when your doctor (or pharmacist in the case of over-the-counter medicine) suggests a medicine, you should always mention any others you are taking regularly, or one you have bought yourself, and ask if it is safe to take them together. Also the effect of some medicines (tranquillisers, for example) is increased by alcohol, and certain anti-depressants react badly with particular foods, such as cheese and Marmite, or some shouldn't be taken with milk, for example. Where necessary, the pharmacist will write detailed warnings on the label, so do be sure to read and follow all instructions exactly.

Along with its needed effects, a medicine may cause side-effects. You should always discuss side-effects with your doctor and let him or her know if you feel unwell or have any unusual discomfort which you do not understand after taking your medicine.

A few people can be allergic to some medicines and if any of the following side-effects develop soon after taking your medicine you should talk to your doctor as soon as possible: sudden wheeziness or tightness in the chest;

swelling of eyelids, face or lip, with or without a lumpy skin rash, or other kind of rash anywhere on the body. Nausea, vomiting or diarrhoea are also among the most common, though usually less serious side-effects. Fortunately, these – and most of the others – will pass and, providing the cause is recognised, the sufferer stops taking the medicine and consults the doctor for advice, all should be well in most cases.

Medicines are available in various forms and absorbed into the bloodstream in different ways – some through the lining membrane in the mouth, some through the stomach lining, and some further down the digestive system in the intestines. So when the directions say 'Take before food' (which means on an empty stomach), or 'Take after food', there is a good reason for this, as food affects the absorption of the medicine.

Almost all medicines and pills will do you harm if taken in too great a quantity or incorrectly. So follow the instructions on the label. Twice the amount won't do you twice as much good, or work any quicker, and could be dangerous.

Never take an analgesic (painkiller) within four hours of having taken one, even if it is of a different type or brand. Tablets or capsules can stick in your throat, so take them with plenty of water while sitting or standing up. Swallow capsules whole, unless you are told to open them.

Medicines can also be given as suppositories or pessaries. If you are prescribed a suppository, unwrap it and follow the instructions. You use it by pushing it into the anus (back passage). Suppositories are popular in many European countries. They are directly absorbed into the bloodstream, so preventing any changes to their active ingredients that might occur if they passed through the digestive system. A pessary is for use in a woman's vagina (front passage). Remember, your pharmacist is an expert on medicines, so always ask for advice if you are not sure what to do.

Medicines can also be given in patch form. The patch is applied to the skin, usually on a hairless area. If you use patches, say for angina, or for hormone replacement therapy, make sure you dispose of them carefully as the old patch will still contain some active ingredient. Ensure children cannot get at them.

Some medicines may cause drowsiness. If affected don't drive or operate machinery and avoid alcoholic drink. Alcohol may change the way your medicine works.

Never put your tablets into another smaller bottle. Always keep medicines in their original containers so you know the labelling is accurate.

If you accidentally take an overdose of your medicine, either get in touch with your doctor immediately, or go to your nearest hospital casualty department. Always take any remaining tablets, the container and the label with you, so that the medicines can be identified correctly.

In the case of some medicines – especially sleeping pills and tranquillisers – an equivalent dose will have a greater effect on the elderly and the dose may have to be adjusted accordingly. This is probably because a person's metabolism tends to slow down with age and their weight sometimes decreases. Children, too, need smaller doses, depending on their age and/or weight and it is important for the doctor or pharmacist to know a child's age before prescribing.

Always finish a course of tablets, however quickly your symptoms may appear to subside, unless your doctor tells you otherwise. Ideally, try to take any tablets at regular intervals, as recommended. Their concentration in the blood will then remain constant and so they will be at their most effective. So if, for example, the directions advise you to take the tablets twice a day do take the tablets every twelve hours, at 8 am and 8 pm, for instance. If the label tells you to take your medicine four times a day it might be helpful to you to divide the day up as 7 am, 12 pm, 6 pm, and finally 12 am so that you don't need to disturb your night's sleep. However, an hour or two 'leeway' should not make too much difference if you need to go to bed earlier and get up later.

If you need to take your medicine every four hours, the necessity of a night-time dosage will depend on the medicine and the illness. Obviously there's no need to put your alarm clock on to wake you in the middle of the night if you're suffering from a nasty bout of flu, but if you have any doubts, check with your GP or pharmacist.

With medicines prescribed long-term, it's usual to see the doctor every three to six months – or at whatever interval he or she suggests – rather than ask the receptionist if you can have a repeat prescription each time. Your doctor may want to check whether you still require that particular treatment, or check your blood pressure, for example, or the dosage may need amending. Bear in mind that symptoms you don't normally suffer, such as nausea or headaches, may be due to tablets you are taking, so don't simply take other remedies to relieve the symptoms without telling your doctor about them first.

If you don't understand a doctor's instructions on a prescribed medicine or exactly how to take it, ask the pharmacist to explain.

I'm often asked by people whether it's worth bothering their doctor, especially if their symptoms turn out to be the result of something inconsequential. But I would say if you are worried about something you should always check it out. As most people don't have any medical training, the only practical criterion you can apply when deciding whether or not to go to the doctor is your own unease and worry.

Your doctor can then either recommend investigation or treatment for worrying new symptoms, or reassure you that there's nothing to be concerned about. Such reassurance for patients is a very straightforward matter and part of a doctor's job, a part that should save you – and him or her – time in the long run.

The Medicines For practical purposes, medicines can be categorised into 3 groups. Prescription Only Medicines (POMs), Pharmacy only medicines (P) and Over the Counter medicines (OTC) – sometimes called the 'General Sales' category.

The first, as the name implies, will only be dispensed routinely upon the prescription of a doctor. The second will regularly be prescribed by a doctor, however they can also be purchased – but only under the watchful, professional eye of a pharmacist.

The third category includes powerful medicines which are, however, 'made safe' for general sale (OTC). This is achieved by being sold only in small pack sizes and with careful instructions on their use. In this way, such excellent remedies as aspirin, for example, can be purchased in pubs, clubs and grocer's shops.

In this book we have included many if not most of the medicines that doctors regularly prescribe, even though they can equally well be obtained, and advice given about their use, from a pharmacist.

There are about 2000 'medicines' which are prescribed under some 5000 names – many of them brand names. So in a book of this size it is not possible to cover them all, or the many different conditions for which they may be prescribed. But I know from my postbag that many if not most of the questions that are regularly asked are covered in this book.

Also, I am grateful to the two to three hundred pharmaceutical companies who have kindly responded to my postal request for the latest details of their products. Inevitably, there will be a few preparations which have been omitted due to nothing more than the practicalities of the task. Rest assured that I will do my best to include them in the first reprint of this book and would welcome a reminder of their absence.

A–Z of Conditions and Illnesses

ACNE AND SPOTS

Acne is a disorder of the sebaceous glands in the skin which causes spots. It's probably one of the most distressing of common skin conditions and it affects almost all youngsters at some time, although severe cases are rare.

Spots usually appear first when the sufferer is anywhere between the ages of 11 and 15, and disappear when he or she is in the mid to late 20s. In rare and depressing cases they can continue into the late 30s. Acne affects the skin on the face, neck, back and chest and is generally worse in men than in women.

Spots normally occur because of an increase in the production of sebum, the skin's normal oily secretion. Sebum keeps the skin moist and supple – without it, the skin would become dry and might even crack. The overproduction of sebum is due to stimulation from a male hormone, androgen, and leads to the shiny skin commonly seen in teenagers. With the increase in this skin grease, the pores in the skin can become blocked and infected by bacteria which thrive on the sebum. This in turn causes spots.

Clearing up acne nearly always needs great perseverance. There is no overnight cure and you may have to persist with treatment for several months at a time. You can buy many preparations including antibacterial skin-washing creams, lotions and soap which can help by reducing bacterial activity in the skin. Antiseptic creams, ointments and soaps can destroy micro-organisms, and abrasives can remove blockages clogging up the skin.

The most common form of treatment available is a keratolytic skin ointment – that means it 'dissolves' the keratin (top layer of the skin) and encourages peeling of the layer of dead and hardened skin cells that form the skin's surface. These ointments – there are a number of different brands – may contain the keratolytics benzoyl peroxide, sulphur or salicylic acid. Benzoyl peroxide and sulphur also have an antibacterial effect.

If you know you have sensitive skin, or have suffered an adverse reaction to other acne preparations in the past, it's worth applying creams or lotions to a small area of skin for the first few days. If your skin seems to tolerate it, you can then treat larger areas.

Keratolytic preparations often cause soreness of the skin, so they are available in different strengths. Benzoyl peroxide, for instance, is likely to cause a mild burning sensation on the first application, as well as a moderate reddening and peeling of the skin during the first few days. Throughout the first few weeks of treatment, most patients will experience a sudden increase in peeling. This isn't harmful and will subside within a day or two if treatment is temporarily discontinued. Then start treatment again and continue while the acne is kept at bay and the other side-effects remain at non-worrying levels.

But if discomfort such as burning, redness or excessive peeling occurs, stop the treatment temporarily or consult your doctor. Patients with a known sensitivity to this active ingredient shouldn't use products which contain it. Preparations containing benzoyl peroxide shouldn't be used for longer than three months at a time.

It's also worth noting that these products may bleach dyed clothing and fabrics, so use them with care.

If keratolytic ointments don't work for you, your doctor may recommend an alternative form of treatment – a cream containing retinoic acid (a vitamin A treatment) or one with an antibiotic, or an antibiotic/anti-inflammatory topical treatment such as Zineryt. This may cause a slight burning sensation or a slight redness of the skin which is due to its alcohol base.

You could be referred to a specialist dermatologist, who may prescribe vitamin A-derivative tablets such as Roaccutane (isotretinoin). Isotretinoin dramatically reduces the formation of grease by the sebaceous glands. It also cuts down on the formation of non-inflamed lesions and the number of bacteria. It also reduces inflammation. It's an effective treatment for severe acne but not without side-effects. It can damage an unborn child if taken during pregnancy. Women shouldn't become pregnant while taking the drug, should practise contraception for at least four weeks before treatment during it and for at least four weeks after it's stopped. This includes even women of child-bearing age with a history of infertility.

Most patients experience drying of the lips, skin (particular on the face) and even eyelids. Up to three in ten develop mild aches and pains of the joints or muscles and 15% have headaches.

If you're female the doctor may suggest the use of a contraceptive pill – either a common one known to be beneficial to the skin or one which, while still having a contraceptive effect, is primarily prescribed for the treatment of acne, Dianette, for example.

Antibiotics can be prescribed for acne. The most common ones to be prescribed are tetracycline or oxytetracycline, usually for a period of six months. Other antibiotics include erythromycin, minocycline, doxycyline and trimethoprim. Antibiotics work in two ways – by reducing the number of bacteria and by reducing the inflammatory response.

This type of treatment is normally thought to be pretty

safe, although rarely an itchy rash can occur which means treatment should be stopped. Other infrequent side-effects include sickness or abdominal pain, or mild diarrhoea.

Remember that if you suffer from acne, you should try to avoid worrying about your spots, as this make them worse. (Easier said than done, I know.) Also restrain yourself from squeezing blackheads and pimples, as this can cause further damage and scarring of the skin, and can also make the spots spread.

Many acne sufferers try not to eat chocolate and other fatty foods, and although there is no real proof that this has any effect on acne, it's worth a try, as a healthy, well-balanced diet with plenty of fresh fruit and vegetables can generally only be good for you. Sunshine can help dry up your spots – but don't overdo it and burn yourself.

Preparations prescribed Actinac, Benzagel 5 & 10, Dalacin T. Topical, Dianette, Ionax Scrub, Nericur Gel 5 & 10, Quinoderm, Roaccutane, Skinoren, Topicycline, Zineryt

ANAEMIA

Anaemia is a red blood cell disorder. It's a reduction in the quantity of oxygen-carrying haemoglobin in the blood and is the most common of all the blood disorders. It has various forms – iron deficiency, pernicious, sickle cell and megaloblastic.

The symptoms of the most common type, iron deficiency, include fatigue, listlessness, apathy and loss of appetite, a sore tongue and inflammation at the sides of the mouth, and dry, brittle nails. It's usually treated by your doctor prescribing a course of iron tablets, or occasionally, iron injections, and she or he will also want to find the underlying cause of the condition. This can be loss of blood due, for example, to heavy periods. Gastric ulcers or piles, where there is heavy hidden blood loss, can also cause anaemia. Some diseases, like rheumatoid arthritis, destroy red blood cells and can in that way cause anaemia. A common and less alarming cause is a diet deficient in iron. When accompanied by a lack of folic acid (needed for normal cell growth) it's called megaloblastic (folate deficient) anaemia; pregnant women and the elderly are particularly vulnerable to this type. Symptoms are a sore tongue, persistent diarrhoea, tingling in the toes and fingers and, in severe cases, the complexion takes on a yellow tint. The treatment is folic acid tablets or, in severe cases, injections.

Bone marrow may be tested to confirm the diagnosis, or other tests may be done to ensure that pernicious anaemia isn't present. This is caused by the bone marrow lacking vitamin B12 or other things needed for blood to form properly. The symptoms are the same as with folate deficient anaemia, but the causes and treatment are different. Pernicious anaemia usually requires injections for life. But provided regular injections are given, this type of anaemia can be controlled.

Anaemia once diagnosed can usually be treated quickly and efficiently without any trauma on the part of the patient. Results are rapid, bringing a swift end to the apathy and tiredness anaemia inflicts. Side-effects of iron supplements can include stomach upsets, nausea, vomiting, diarrhoea or constipation. Iron supplements may also be prescribed as a preventive measure. It helps, too, to eat a healthy diet particularly one which is iron- and vitamin-B-rich and includes plenty of green leafy vegetables, fish, red meat, liver and watercress. Eating some foods together helps the absorption of iron – eating red meat with spinach or a drink of fresh orange juice which is rich in vitamin C.

Preparations prescribed Fergon, Ferrocontin Continus Tablets, Ferromyn Elixir, Niferex Elixir, Niferex-150, Slow-Fe

ANAL ITCHING

Itching around the anus (back passage) is a common problem and is known medically as *pruritis ani*. It is slightly more common in men and people often put up with it for years, trying various self-help remedies (which may do more harm than good) because they are too embarrassed to consult their doctor. *Pruritis ani* can be a symptom of an underlying condition, such as diabetes, or an infection, for which treatment is needed, so if you have this kind of itching, it really is important to be examined by a doctor.

Often, however, the condition is brought about by the sufferer him or herself. For instance, research has shown that people who tend to worry about their bowels and take laxatives to keep them regular, are particularly prone. The laxatives, especially liquid paraffin, may cause leakage, or several bowel movements a day. Excessive amounts of high fibre foods can have the same effect. Frequent wiping or washing then becomes necessary and this can soon chafe the skin and set up a constant irritation. Some people become obsessed about disinfecting or deodorising the area, using quite strong solutions that can make matters worse. Laxity of the anal sphincter (the normally tight band of muscle at the exit) can also lead to leakage and consequent irritation. So too can frequent straining to pass a motion, or increased pressure within the rectum, due to piles, for example (see page 129).

Other conditions that can lead to a rectal discharge and irritation include an anal fissure or fistula, Crohn's disease (see page 44), genital warts and a polyp – a small, benign growth.

A vaginal discharge due to an infection, such as trichomonas, can also affect the anal region as well as the vulval and cause pruritus.

The anal area, being warm and moist, is prone to other infections, such as the fungus which also causes the vaginal thrush (see page 151) that many women suffer from. This infection is more likely to thrive in overweight people whose skin often becomes chafed but an anti-fungal cream prescribed by the doctor usually clears up the infection quickly. Overweight people also tend to sweat more which adds to any irritation, as the anal skin is richly supplied with itch spots which are aggravated by warmth. A cool bath or bidet will usually relieve the itching or at night, when the itching is often worst, bathing the area with a damp sponge can be very soothing.

Threadworms are another cause (see page 164) or a much rarer infestation, scabies, may be the cause, too, (see page 143). Skin conditions, such as eczema and psoriasis, can cause irritation around the anus. Sometimes it will occur following a course of antibiotics. Some people are sensitive to soaps, deodorants and biological washing powders and these can lead to a dermatitis and recurrent episodes of intense itching. It will be a question of trial and error to see which, if any, is affecting you. It often helps to shave the area, as this reduces chafing, and cotton underpants are best. Calamine lotion should also be soothing. After a bowel movement, bathe the area with luke warm water, with no antiseptics added. Avoid scratching, if at all possible, and do not rub in creams or ointments too vigorously.

As you can see, there are many possible causes for this kind of itching so do consult your doctor for a definite diagnosis and advice as the condition can be made worse if, say, the wrong type of cream is used. Most of the problems settle down with suitable treatment perhaps a cream such as Proctosedyl which contains a mild topical steroid such as hydrocortisone to ease itching and inflammation and a local anaesthetic to relieve pain; or a cream containing hydrocortisone and an anti-fungal agent such as Canesten HC. Just occasionally symptoms persist and then referral to a specialist will usually be recommended.

Preparations prescribed Anacal, Anugesic HC, Gentisone HC Cream/Ointment, Proctofoam HC, Proctosedyl, Scheriproct Ointment and Suppositories, Timodine, Ultraproct, Xylocaine, Xyloproct

ANGINA

Angina (*angina pectoris*) is attacks of chest pain due to reduction of the flow of blood through the coronary arteries which supply the heart muscle. Pain can also be experienced in the arm or neck. For most people the main cause of the condition is the narrowing of the coronary arteries, as the fatty substance atheroma is laid down just below the inner lining of the coronary blood vessels. As a result, less blood is able to get to the heart muscle, less quickly than usual, because of the 'pinched' flow.

If only one of the three main coronary arteries is pinched, then angioplasty can bring remarkable relief. This, the blowing up of a 'balloon' in the coronary artery, opens up the restriction, so the blood can flow normally again. A heart bypass operation (where a blood vessel from another part of the body bypasses the artery) is another surgical technique.

In some families, angina and heart problems are more common than most. Usually, this means that they have a much higher level of cholesterol – fat – in their blood than is normal. This condition is known as familial hyperlipidaemia. When it is present, both men and women may suffer from angina or heart attacks in their early 30s.

When one member of the family is discovered to have excessively high levels of cholesterol, perhaps after a heart attack, the other members of the family will be offered advice on lifestyle, but will also be prescribed medicines which lower the blood concentration of cholesterol.

Angina symptoms can be relieved with drugs – nitrates, beta-blockers and calcium antagonists. Nitrates such as glyceryl trinitrate (Nitrocontin Continus) or isorbide dinitrate (Sorbichew), for example, are vasodilators – they relax the muscles in the walls of the coronary arteries (and arteries elsewhere in the body) allowing more blood to flow to the heart's muscle, and so relieve the pain.

Beta-blockers (atenolol (Tenormin) for example) act on the nerves which control circulation while calcium antagonists (nifedipine (Adalat) for example) alter the way minerals enter and leave the body cells.

Side-effects of medicines to treat angina can include headache, dizziness, flushing, cold hands and feet, sleep disturbance, tiredness or stomach upsets.

As well as tablets, patches can now be used to treat angina. They contain glyceryl trinitrate (Transiderm-Nitro, or Deponit 5 & 10). The patches release the medicine through the skin and into the blood vessels. They reduce the heart's need for oxygen and also increase blood supply to the heart which helps stop the pain of angina. The patches can be placed on the front or side of the chest, the upper abdomen or upper arm. Reddening of the skin can be eased by putting a patch in a different place each day.

Preparations prescribed Adalat, Adizem, Betaloc, Betaloc SA, Beta Prograne, Blocadren, Cardinol, Deponit, Emcor, Emcor LS, Geangin, Glytrin Spray, Imdur, Inderal, Inderal LA/Half-Inderal LA, Lopresor, Lopresor SR, Monit LS, Mycardol, Nitrocontin Continus Tablets, Nitro-Dur, Percutol, Sectral, Slow-Trasicor, Sorbitrate, Sorbichew, Sorbid, Tenif, Tenormin, Tildiem, Tildiem Retard 90 and 120, Totamol, Transiderm-Nitro, Trasicor, Univer, Visken

ANTIBIOTICS

Penicillin was the first antibiotic to be introduced and has been in use for more than 50 years. There are now many different groups of antibiotics and within those groups several different types. The groups include penicillins, cephalosporins, tetracyclines, macrolides, quinolones, sulphonamides, aminoglycosides and lincosamides among others.

Antibiotics are used frequently to treat a wide range of infections such as upper respiratory tract infections (tonsillitis, pharyngitis, laryngitis, sinusitis, for example); lower respiratory tract infections including acute and chronic bronchitis and pneumonia; secondary infections in colds and influenza; tuberculosis and to help stop the spread of some forms of meningitis; ear infections; oral infections, for example, gingivitis; eye, skin and soft tissue infections and genito-urinary infections including cystitis and gonorrhoea – to name but a few!

Antibiotics are chemicals which work, in general, by stopping the growth of micro-organisms and then destroying them. The wide range of antibiotics available is testimony to the wide range of micro-organisms that exist – and antibiotics are not effective against all micro-organisms. Some are effective for some problems, others for other problems, but remember that antibiotics are not effective against virus infections.

Amoxycillin, Erythromycin, Tetracycline and Penicillin are most GPs stand-bys.

Antibiotics which come under the penicillins (often with the name ... cillin) should not be taken by people who are allergic to penicillin. Penicillins are the largest group of antibiotics and side-effects are not that common. When side-effects are experienced they are usually mild and fairly short-lived. They may include diarrhoea, indigestion or, more often, a blotchy rash – those suffering from glandular fever may develop a rash if they take a penicillin, for example, so these are avoided when an antibiotic is needed.

Cephalosporins can cause diarrhoea, nausea, vomiting and skin rashes. Tetracyclines can cause thrush or diarrhoea. Children's teeth can be stained by these medicines so they are avoided for children and in women known to be pregnant since the future teeth of the developing baby may be affected.

Macrolides (erythromycin is the main one in this group) is a widely used and very effective antibiotic. It can cause nausea and stomach upsets.

I regularly receive letters which go something like this: 'I've been put on a course of antibiotics for a throat infection and feel generally miserable. A friend says this could be a side-effect of the medicine. Should I stop taking the antibiotics?' The answer is that you probably shouldn't stop taking them immediately as, unlike many medicines, antibiotics don't treat the symptoms of the illness directly. The body itself does this as the antibiotics destroy the invading germs. Consequently, while the antibiotics are taking their time to work, many people will continue to feel ill and may assume this is a side-effect. Also, people are often a bit in awe of antibiotics and many assume such powerful cures must have strong side-effects, so they feel strange as a result. Having said this, some people genuinely do have a strong reaction to some antibiotics, in the same way some people react to certain foods.

These side-effects, as I've already mentioned, include vomiting, a rash, puffiness of the tissues, or breathlessness. However, unless you have one of these, or another apparent side-effect which is severe, it would be better to consult your doctor or pharmacist before stopping.

Some people, especially the older generation will often say to me 'the antibiotics are too strong for me'. This is because they remember the days when the antibiotics were first introduced. They revolutionised the treament of bacterial infection and stopped people dying as a result. What my readers or patients are really saying is that they feel different while taking them, perhaps a little sick or off their food. In most cases, it is safe for them to make the choice not to take them, unless they have a life threatening condition.

Another worry about antibiotics troubles many parents, particularly if their children have frequently had bouts of colds, sore throats and coughs, with seemingly constant prescriptions for antibiotics. The worry is that the antibiotics could prevent their bodies from producing their own antibodies, and that the children would be more susceptible to illness as a result.

But I doubt it. For one thing, the family doctor has probably waited for signs of bacterial infection before prescribing antibiotics. You see, the bulk of such infections are likely to be due to viruses, and antibiotics are not effective against these – so they will have been overcome by your children's self-grown antibodies, anyway.

What antibiotics can do is destroy secondary invaders – the bacteria that are more able to catch hold when tissues are already disturbed by virus infection. Their presence will start the production of natural antibodies, whether or not they are subsequently destroyed by the antibiotics.

When more than one young child is in the house throughout the winter, any infection introduced by one of them can readily spread around. Outdoor activities and opening the windows, whenever possible and it's not too cold out, will keep viruses at bay.

Preparations prescribed Amoxycillin, Amfipen, Augmentin, Bactrim, Ceporex, Chloromycetin, Erymax, Erythroped, Galenamox, Galfloxin, Imperacin, Klaricid, Monotrim, Nordox, Orelox, Septrin, Stafoxil, Tarivid, Zinnat

ANXIETY

The symptoms of anxiety, a mixture of physical and emotional symptoms such as listlessness, headaches, nervousness and irritability, depression – most often at night – dizziness, panic or palpitations, insomnia, and gastric upsets, are due to over-activity of our autonomous nervous system – the one over which we have little or no control.

The control that is needed is the ability to relax tense muscles and to calm the whole mind. This, in turn, calms other 'wires'. It's rather like calming the switchboard operators at a manual telephone exchange and so allowing everyone's calls to be put through efficiently.

Benzodiazepines (tranquillisers) may be given because they calm anxiety, help induce sleep and muscle relaxation. Examples are diazepam, clorazepate dipotassium, lorazepam. They are useful and effective drugs but must be used with extreme care, always in the lowest dose possible. They are usually recommended for short-term use of approximately two to four weeks and only then when anxiety is moderate to severe. In other words, when it's such strong anxiety it's disabling or subjecting a person to unacceptable distress. Long-term treatment with benzodiazepines can lead to dependence and withdrawal symptoms in certain patients.

Patients taking this type of medicine should be carefully monitored and routine repeat prescriptions should be avoided. Treatment should always be withdrawn gradually to reduce the risk of withdrawal symptoms developing.

Side-effects can include drowsiness, light-headedness, ataxia, confusion, vertigo, stomach upsets, as well as low blood pressure, visual disturbances and skin rashes.

Beta-blockers (e.g. propranolol or oxprenolol) can sometimes be prescribed to help anxiety states. These drugs help to reduce the physical symptoms sufferers can find so distressing, such as sweating and tremors. Side-effects are usually mild and short-lived and include cold hands and feet, nausea, diarrhoea, lassitude and muscle fatigue.

Buspirone (Buspar) is a newer drug (it's an azapirone) and is used for the short-term treatment of anxiety disorders. It's said to have fewer side-effects and less chance of being abused than the benzodiazepines. The most likely side-effects are dizziness, light-headedness, excitement, headache and nausea.

Most people suffering from anxiety are likely to be successfully treated by their GP – only a minority will need specialist psychiatric help. Confiding in a friend or relative about something worrying can help. Or just trying to sit down and think of the problems that are making you anxious and trying to find ways of resolving them. Regular exercise can help relieve tension. This may be because exercise induces the body to release its natural tranquillisers, the hormones called endorphins.

Preparations prescribed Beta Prograne, Buspar, chlordiazepoxide, diazepam, Inderal, Inderal LA/Half-Inderal LA, lorazepam, oxazepam, Oxypertine, Stemetil, Stemetil Eff, Trancopal

ARTHRITIS

Arthritis refers to something much more than an aching pain, and being told you have it could mean one of a large number of different things. There are many, many types of arthritis, from osteoarthritis through to reactive arthritis – which can be a relatively short-lived type of inflammation of the joints after a viral infection such as glandular fever or German measles (rubella arthritis). Some people are hardly aware of their arthritis, while other find everyday life an uphill struggle. Arthritis can be extremely painful and debilitating.

The most common form is osteoarthritis, which usually affects the over-50s, and not many people can escape some degree of it in their old age. The disease causes so much pain because it damages joint surfaces – thus inhibiting the painless and proper use of the joint. When osteoarthritis develops, the protective, shock-absorbing rubbery substance called cartilage, which covers the ends of the bones at the joints to protect them, becomes worn and rough and is almost 'rubbed away'. In places it splits so that the bone underneath thickens and spreads out, enlarging the joint. It mainly affects the weight-bearing joints and those in constant use such as knees, hips, spine and fingers. Sometimes the neck and lower back are involved. Shoulders are commonly the last to be affected.

Rheumatoid arthritis, although not as common as osteoarthritis, can be far more disabling. An inflammatory disease which makes joints stiff, painful and swollen, it can cause crippling joint damage and the deformities caused are often more severe than those in other forms of arthritis. It's the most common type of severe arthritis in people below the age of 50. It's a progressive form of arthritis which leads to a gradual deterioration in the affected joints. About a third of patients experience severe disability.

Rheumatoid arthritis tends to strike the smaller joints, for example, in the hands, feet and wrist. The fingers can also become swollen and lumpy. The disease may not progress further, or it can develop in larger joints, such as the knees, ankles, elbows, wrists, shoulders and hips.

Drugs are used effectively to treat arthritis by greatly reducing pain and inflammation. But sometimes hitting on the right drug for you is a question of trial and error – what's acceptable to one person may not suit another.

There are many types of non-steroidal anti-inflammatory drugs available. They work by inhibiting the production of prostaglandins, which pass on pain signals to the brain. Examples of ones used in the treatment of arthritis are mild pain-relievers like aspirin or ibuprofen (Nurofen, Brufen), or drugs such as naproxen (Naprosyn, for example), mefenamic acid (Ponstan) and indomethacin (Indocid or Flexin, for instance). Indomethacin is one of the most popular and widely prescribed drugs in the treatment of arthritis as it seems to be effective time and again. Analgesics are also used for pain relief, although they don't help inflammation – examples are paracetamol and the opiate codeine. Paracetamol can be useful when a person is intolerant of aspirin.

The most common side-effects of non-steroidal anti-inflammatory drugs include nausea, vomiting, heartburn or indigestion. Naproxen can cause gastrointestinal disorders, as can mefenamic acid. Indomethacin commonly causes gastrointestinal disturbances, headaches, drowsiness and even depression. Combination medicines such as Arthrotec contain a NSAID preparation as well as another which quietens any gastric irritation that this may cause.

Anti-rheumatic drugs help stop or slow down the disease process although why they do so is not entirely understood. They work more slowly than anti-inflammatory drugs and sometimes it takes quite a while before any benefit is noticed. Examples of these are gold-based drugs – sodium aurothiomalate (Myocrisin) and auranofin (Ridaura), penicillamine (Pendramine, for example) and more recently sulphasalazine (Salazopyrin), the anti-malarial drug chloroquine (Avloclor, for example) and also immunosuppressives like methotrexate (Arthitrex, for example). Immunosuppressives work by suppressing cells thought to cause the damage in arthritis and are used only when absolutely necessary because of their effects on blood in particular.

These types of drugs are used for serious forms of arthritis and unfortunately do often cause unpleasant side-effects. Blood, kidneys and your liver will need to be monitored for signs of toxicity. Gold-based drugs cause diarrhoea and skin rash and affect the kidneys and blood cells. Penicillamine can cause allergic rashes and itching, gastrointestinal disturbances and loss of taste. Sulphasalazine (particularly with higher doses) can cause nausea, vomiting, loss of appetite, ringing in the ears, headache and joint pain. Orange or yellow discoloration of the urine can occur. Chloroquine may cause nausea, diarrhoea and vomiting and can eventually affect the eyes by the formation of corneal deposits.

Steroids (corticosteroid drugs) can also be used effectively to reduce inflammation. (see Steroids page 149). An example is methylprednisolone (Medrone).

Preparations prescribed Arthitrex, Arthrotec, Arthroxen, Avloclor, Brufen, Caprin, Clinoril, Codafen Continus, Cytotec, Decadron, Diclomax Retard, Disalcid, Dolobid, Emflex, Flexin, Fortagesic, Indocid, Lodine, Mobiflex, Motrin, Myocrisin, Napratec, Naprosyn, Pendramine, Plaquenil, Ponstan, Pranoxen, Prednesol, Relifex, Rheumox, Ridaura, Salazopyrin, Surgam, Voltarol, Zantac

ASTHMA

The condition causes a recurrent cough, tightness of the chest or a wheeze, or all three. It's an inflammatory condition that causes a swelling of the lining membrane of the breathing tubes, which constricts them. Also, the very small muscles in these tubes contract, narrowing them further. In Britain, about 2,000 people a year die, and more end up brain-damaged, as a result of a serious asthma attack. More than one in ten of us suffer from asthma – and it seems to be on the increase. No one really knows why, but specialists may be spotting it more often, bringing earlier relief. Symptoms – a frequent 'tightness', a shortness of breath, a wheeze or a cough – are worse sometimes than at other times. And it's this variable obstruction to the lungs' airways which is the true characteristic of asthma.

Trigger factors can include an allergy – one of the most common causes of asthma. The most common allergens are pollens, house-dust mites and animals. Chest infections can trigger asthma. In adults, attacks are not necessarily caused by an allergy, but by over-reaction of the lung-lining tissues to the cold, for example, or to exercise. In someone who already has asthma, worry and anxiety and pressure at work or at home can make asthma worse.

Asthma is surprisingly common and can be treated easily and effectively. If asthma is diagnosed, your doctor will probably prescribe an inhaler. Medicines are given to help prevent the symptoms occurring or to give relief when you have symptoms.

The medicines used to treat asthma include bronchodilators (airway openers) and inhaled steroids. The major bronchodilators are salbutamol (Ventolin, for example) and terbutaline (Bricanyl), best taken by inhaler or in the form of an aerosol mist by a nebuliser, because this means that small amounts of medicine reach the airways quickly to relax muscle spasm. You can also be prescribed bronchodilators in tablet or syrup form. Most common side-effects of salbutamol include mild muscle tremor (usually the hands), anxiety and restlessness. Terbutaline produces low side-effects at recommended doses but these include tremor, cramp and palpitations.

Theophylline is another kind of bronchodilator prescribed in capsule, tablet or syrup form and relaxes bronchial muscles. (Lasma, for example). Most common side-effects include nausea or vomiting.

Inhaled steroids (Becloforte, for instance) are effective as they help damp down the irritability of the airways. In standard doses there are relatively few side-effects because of the small size of the doses involved and because, when inhaled, the medicine goes straight to the airways. This lowers the risk of the medicine affecting any other part of the body. Sometimes patients develop a mild throat infection, and occasionally others do find that their voice becomes husky. It might help to rinse your mouth thoroughly with water after using such a medicine.

Flixotide is a recently introduced preparation which is claimed to have twice the effect with virtually no absorption through the airway lining, so reducing the body dose still further.

Sodium cromoglycate (Intal, for example) is also used to prevent symptoms of asthma. It may prevent the release of certain chemicals in the airways which cause spasm. It can also cause throat irritation, coughing and brief bronchospasm. Steroid tablets (Medrone, for example) may be needed for severe asthma.

People with asthma have airways which have become over-sensitive. So if you suffer from asthma and know what triggers an attack, do try to avoid that trigger. Try to keep your house as free from dust as possible. Even though exercise can bring on wheezing, moderate exercise should be undertaken, especially in children. Using a bronchodilator drug before exercise helps to prevent an attack. Most asthmatics find that swimming is a helpful form of exercise. Always keep your drugs close at hand. If you feel your asthma is getting worryingly worse, you should contact your doctor.

Preparations prescribed Aerobec, Aerolin, Alupent, Becloforte, Becotide, Berotec, Bricanyl, Choledyl, Duovent, Exirel, Flixotide Diskhaler, Lasma, Medihaler, Medrone, Nuelin, Oxivent, Phyllocontin, Prednesol, Pro-Vent, Pulmadil Inhaler, Pulmicort, Serevent, Theo-dur, Uniphyllin, Ventide, Ventolin, Zaditen

ATHLETE'S FOOT

Athlete's foot (*tinea pedis*) is a fungal infection of the skin which thrives in warm, wet conditions. The skin between the toes becomes red, soggy, itchy, flaky and sometimes smelly. It's not very common in children but is a frequent problem for adolescents and sporty young men and women who use communal changing rooms. The condition will persist until it's treated and, as other people can be infected, prompt attention is required.

Treatment is fairly straightforward. If you suffer from athlete's foot – or as a precaution against it – you should ensure your feet are kept dry. 'Air' them as often as possible, wash them frequently, particularly during hot weather, change socks or stockings daily and avoid walking barefoot in public changing rooms. If you have to use a changing room or communal shower, try wearing sandals to avoid any risk of infection from the floor.

Antifungal creams, sprays or powders are usually very effective. They mainly contain antifungal drugs such as tolnaftate, undecenoic acid, miconazole, dichlorophen or zinc undecenoate and need to be used morning and night after thoroughly washing your feet (always use your own flannel and towel) and removing any loose skin. Rub creams or sprays into and around affected skin. Sprinkle powder liberally on to feet, particularly between the toes. It's helpful, too, to dust socks and the insides of shoes before wearing them. Unless the instructions on your medicine advise you differently, continue treatment for a week after all signs of infection have disappeared.

If the condition doesn't clear up in a week or so, you may need a stronger antifungal agent than those available over the counter. Consult your doctor who may prescribe a medicine such as Lamisil Cream (terbinafine). For severe infections you could be prescribed an oral anti-fungal agent such as Lamisil (terbinafine). This type of treatment can cause mild to moderate and short-lived side-effects such as gastrointestinal symptoms or allergic skin reactions.

Preparations prescribed Exelderm, Lamisil, Loceryl, Masnoderm, Nizoral, Polyfax, Sporanox, Tinaderm-M Cream, Tineafax Cream or Powder

BACK PAIN

Back pain is an extremely common problem – it can affect as many as two out of three people. It can rarely be ignored and often doesn't provoke the sympathy and understanding that it should, probably because pain is such a subjective thing, and also since back problems can be so varied and complex.

That's because the spine stretches from the bottom of your skull to your buttocks and is made up of 24 vertebrae and 110 joints. It surrounds and protects the spinal cord, the main means of nerve communication between all parts of the body and the brain. There's a network of nerves, each one linked to the spinal cord between the vertebrae.

Discs lie between each vertebra to cushion them as the spine moves and to serve as shock absorbers. Then there's a complicated network of muscles and ligaments holding the whole lot together – so you can see why there's so much scope for trouble.

The most common causes of back pain are sprains, strains or a tear in one of the ligaments or muscles. Another common cause is a mechanical failure of some part of the structure of the spine leading to a bone becoming slightly displaced. Sciatica is a common form of low back pain. This is an inflammation of the sciatic nerve – the largest nerve in the body – often triggered by bending from the waist instead of from the knees, particularly when lifting a heavy object and twisting the body at the same time. Pain is also felt down the back of the thigh, or front of the leg.

About one in 200 people suffer the severe pain of a slipped disc (prolapsed disc to use the correct term). The discs don't actually slip out but when subjected to too much stress 'burst' (prolapse) enabling some of the soft inner pulp to leak out or bulge (herniate), pressing on surrounding nerves and tissues and causing great pain. Among other causes of back pain are arthritis and osteoporosis (bone thinning).

It's thought that as many as one and a half million people in the UK could be suffering some degree of back pain at any one time. And most cases improve with no more than staying in bed and taking things easy and/or painkilling drugs.

Yet for some people this doesn't seem a sufficient treatment. So often these days people find it difficult to relax and do nothing – and even feel guilty about it. In fact, bed rest is helpful, particularly when the cause of the pain is a sprain, strain or tear (as most are). The injured area does need a period of rest to make it easier for healing to get underway. But don't stay in bed for too long – some experts believe that sufferers should get up and start moving about as soon as the pain eases enough to be able to do so.

Initial treatment for back trouble usually involves dealing with the pain. Aspirin and other non-steroidal anti-inflammatory drugs like ibuprofen (Nurofen, Proflex, Inoven, for example) and naproxen (Naprosyn, for example) which can ease pain as well as reducing stiffness and inflammation can be helpful.

Ibuprofen (also available in a gel form called Ibugel, Ibuleve or Ibuleve Sports Gel) is a popular choice. It's thought to work by blocking the enzyme needed for the production of prostaglandins, which would pass on pain signals to the brain. Prostaglandins also cause inflammation, heat and swelling which makes you feel even worse and can inhibit movement. Indomethacin, another non-steroidal anti-inflammatory drug used in the treatment of arthritis, can sometimes be prescribed for back pain, as can muscle relaxants such as diazepam or methocarbamol (Robaxin).

Paracetamol, or combined analgesics – co-codamol, co-proxamol, co-dydramol – are often prescribed, depending on the intensity of your pain but these won't help reduce inflammation. Other painkillers contain mixtures of paracetamol and codeine, such as Solpadeine, or paracetamol, aspirin and codeine in the case of Veganin, are available over-the-counter. There are other products on the market aimed at back pain, such as Doan's, which contains paracetamol and sodium salicylate, a mild pain reliever.

Your doctor may also prescribe one of the topical non-steroidal anti-inflammatory drugs like Feldene Gel, or

Movelat or Traxam. These can be helpful in relieving pain and inflammation.

You may also be prescribed one of the many counter-irritants, like Algipan containing methyl nicotinate, which make the skin redden and warm, so easing muscular pain and stiffness. Another possibility is a cream like Transvasin, containing benzocaine, a local anaesthetic. There are many rubs available over the counter like the Deep Heat range, for example.

Preparations prescribed Algesal, Cremalgin Balm, Diclomax Retard, Disalcid, Equagesic, Feldene, Indocid, Intralgin, Motrin, Movelat, Naprosyn, Norflex Injection, Orudis, Pranoxen Continus, Proflex, Remedeine, Robaxin 750, Surgam, Traxam, Voltarol

BACTERIAL SKIN INFECTIONS

Bacterial skin infections can include impetigo (a highly contagious skin problem which mainly affects children), and folliculitis – when a slightly more virulent germ than usual gets established in the hair follicle. It is then able to spread so that it can settle in other hair follicles. It's likely that the germs are hardly more harmful than the usual germs on the skin, but they have just become established and entrenched. They not only live in hair follicles but also breed in the warm and moist places in the body, just inside the nose and in the cheeks of the bottom, for example. Although it may sound odd, to cure the condition you need to rid the body of these nests of germs. Boils – sometimes called furuncles – are usually due to a bacterial infections of the skin and are extremely painful. A boil usually starts in and around a hair follicle where skin cells are destroyed by bacteria. Pus then develops, building up such pressure that the boil can burst.

Your doctor may prescribe an ointment whose active ingredient is an antibiotic such as mupirocin (Bactroban), which can kill the bacteria responsible for the majority of superficial skin infections, for example *staphylococcus aureus*. Alternatively an ointment or cream containing gentamicin (Cidomycin, Genticin) may be prescribed. This is a wide-spectrum antibiotic recommended for the treatment of bacterial skin infections and other skin problems such as dermatitis or burns which have become infected. Sometimes you'll need to take a course of antibiotic tablets, pencillin, flucloxacillin or cloxacillin for example.

Topical antibacterial medicines can sometimes sting, burn or cause itching sensations when they are applied. When such ointments are used on the face, extra care should be taken to avoid getting any ointment in your eyes.

Preparations prescribed Bactroban, Cicatrin, Cidomycin, Floxapen, Genticin, Naseptin, Polyfax, Soframycin, Quinoderm

BITES AND STINGS

Creatures that sting do so to protect themselves, insects that bite do so to feed. With mosquitoes, midges and horseflies it is only the female that bites; she needs the blood that a good bite gives her in order to rear her young – no consolation to us as we scratch away!

But whether the attack takes the form of a bite or a sting, the result is the same – a hot, red, swollen, itchy area and sometimes, more serious consequences. In the case of a sting, the symptoms are the result of the body's reaction to the poison injected; with a bite, they are due to anti-clotting substance in the insect's saliva which it injects to make the blood flow more easily as it feeds. Although it is not poisonous, this substance can provoke an allergic-type response around the bite and occasionally throughout the body. Fortunately, mosquitoes in Britain do not carry disease.

When you are bitten early in the season, you're more likely to react and find yourself scratching than later on in the summer. This is because your body gradually develops some tolerance, particularly to your local gnats and midges. However this will not help you when you visit a different area and get bitten by an unfamiliar species!

Some people seem to be more attractive to biting insects than others and individuals differ in how much they react. In general, though, insect-repellents should protect you for about two hours and, if you are bitten, iced water or witch-hazel, calamine lotion or soothing antiseptic creams available from the chemist will usually calm the irritation. Other over-the-counter remedies tend to be antihistamine medicines or creams, made specifically for bites and stings, to combat any allergic reactions. They can also reduce more severe swelling and irritation and some contain local anaesthetics to ease pain or irritation.

For insect bite reactions your doctor may prescribe creams or ointments containing the mild topical corticosteroid hydrocortisone, (Mildison Lipocream for example) or a local anaesthetic such as lignocaine (Xylocaine). Also for mild, local allergic reactions to insect bites, antihistamine tablets may be prescribed (see HAY FEVER page 81).

However, a few people develop an allergy to wasp or bee stings and can then have an extreme, even life-threatening reaction which may come on only seconds after the sting. The sufferer may feel dizzy and sick, have a runny, itchy nose and eyes and develop a rash. Their limbs may swell, they may have difficulty breathing and even lose consciousness. If any of these symptoms occurs after being stung, it is essential to get to a hospital with an accident and emergency unit (casualty department) or to a doctor immediately.

Similarly, for stings in the mouth, multiple stings or if a child under the age of two is stung, it is best to seek medical advice without delay.

Swimming can be a risky business in some waters. If you are stung by a jellyfish you may not feel it at the time but if you develop a painful, swollen area on your body and perhaps a temperature after swimming in the sea, do consult a doctor.

Stinging fish exist even around the British coast and if you tread on one you will certainly know it – the pain is excruciating. The best treatment is to immerse the stung part in very hot but not scalding water. This will quickly deactivate the venom.

Snake bites in Britain are unlikely to be too serious – the adder is our only venomous snake – but measures such as sucking the wound or making an incision with a razor blade to squeeze out the venom can do more harm than good. It's best to immobilise the bitten limb with a splint or sling and take the person straight to hospital.

For a bee sting, remove the sting with a fingernail by scraping it out sideways and in the direction the sting is pointing outwards, rather than pinching and pulling it out, as this can squeeze the remaining venom into the skin. To counteract the acid in a bee sting, apply ice-cold water containing a little bicarbonate of soda. Wasp stings are alkaline, so bathe them with a little vinegar in ice-cold water. A wasp doesn't leave its sting behind, just a chemical irritant.

Take care when you're out and about. Don't use perfume, hair sprays or aftershave when bees or wasps are around, as they can be attracted by the scent. Bright colours may also attract insects, so wear pale clothes that cover your arms and legs against gnats and midges, especially if you are prone to insect bites. Examine food and sweet drinks before putting them in your mouth and wipe food from your lips if eating out of doors. Don't panic if bees or wasps buzz around you and don't hit out at them. Either ignore them or walk away. And a final safeguard – wear shoes in the garden and when paddling – particularly in rock pools.

Preparations prescribed Hydrocortisyl, Mildison Lipocream, Periactin, Piriton Tablets/Injection, Primalan, Sofra-tulle, Xylocaine

BRONCHITIS

Fortunately, most people who suffer from acute bronchitis (inflammation of the airways connecting the windpipe to the lungs) will not have a continuing problem. Most attacks of bronchitis follow an infection of the lining membranes in the nose, throat or sinuses – what doctors call an upper respiratory tract infection. This is because once a cold, influenza or a respiratory virus invades the nose and upper membranes, it can so easily extend its invasion downwards and affect the main breathing tubes. These airways are called the bronchi.

Indeed, if the germ is a particularly virulent one, or if the sufferer's defences are low, then it can spread down into the smaller tubes, the bronchioles, often causing bronchiolitis. Sometimes it even infects the final breathing membrane, when it causes pneumonia. At that stage, because there is so much of that membrane (if spread out it could cover several table-tennis tables), it is a real assault upon the body's defences. That's why pneumonia, especially, is treated with antibiotics. Before these were available, many attacks of pneumonia ended in tragedy. Antibiotics can be given – for example, ampicillin, amoxycillin, pivampicillin, erythromycin, and the tetracyclines.

Antibiotics may be given to adults with chronic bronchitis (congestion and inflammation of the bronchial tubes) who are suffering an acute attack. It is most important for smokers with chronic bronchitis to stop smoking. In severe cases, a bronchodilator drug is given to widen the airways, helping to overcome breathlessness. Cough mixtures and physiotherapy can help to clear the phlegm. See also ASTHMA (page 25) for modes of treatment.

Preparations prescribed Alupent, Atrovent, Bricanyl, Berotec, Duovent, Franol, Franol Plus, Lasma, Medihaler, Miraxid, Nuelin, Phyllocontin, Pulmadil, Salbulin, Uniphyllin, Ventolin

CATARRH

See COLD, THE COMMON page 37

CHICKENPOX

Chickenpox is a common disease. It's contagious and is caused by a virus called herpes zoster. The same virus also causes shingles. More often than not chickenpox is caught in childhood when it's less severe than in adulthood. And once you've caught it you'll be immune to it. Although having said that, the virus can lie dormant and later on in life can cause shingles (see page 144).

You'll notice chickenpox developing when a rash of small, red spots appears on the body and then spreads to the arms, legs, face and head. The spots change to watery blisters that either burst or shrivel up and crust over. The virus can make you feel generally unwell and there may be a raised temperature. A soothing cream such as calamine lotion helps reduce the itchiness. Try not to scratch as this can cause infection. Paracetamol – particularly for children – will help lower any raised temperature. A medicine such as Periactin (cyproheptadine hydrochloride) may be prescribed. This acts upon the irritant chemicals released into the tissues local to the spots. It can soothe the itching of chickenpox and also gently sedates the sufferer. Anti-histamine medicines supplied by your pharmacist may also bring relief.

Preparation prescribed: Panadol Baby and Infant Suspension (see also PAINKILLERS page 121), Periactin

COLD, THE COMMON
also known as Coryza

The common cold is a virus infection that is spread from one person to another by droplet infection – the usually unseen aerosol of droplets blown into the air when someone with a cold breathes out but especially when they cough or sneeze.

About a hundred different viruses have been shown to cause the symptoms of a cold. This is one of the reasons why we continue to catch them, since even if we build up our anti-bodies to the cold germ that we've just had, another can come along and immediately take hold should we breathe in a sufficiently large number from another sufferer. Also, the anti-bodies that we do produce are short lived. Consequently, the same virus can cause another cold very shortly afterwards if we get re-infected with it.

The main symptoms are an unpleasant tingling sensation in the nose and throat, sneezing, coughing and a temperature in the worst cases – though usually only raised by a degree or so Centigrade.

A cold tends to go of its own accord in a few days. Aspirin or paracetamol in an adult and paracetamol in a child will relieve the worst of the symptoms and help to bring the temperature back to normal.

Sinus Pain, Nasal Congestion and Catarrh

Nasal congestion and catarrh – nasal discharge, or phlegm in the throat – are usually present for a few days during and after many infections of the nose and sinuses, especially the common cold. The combination is a harmless but annoying problem that can be stubborn to shift and can also result in deafness if it builds up in the eustachian tubes (the tubes on either side at the back of the nose and throat), which lead to the ears.

One of the best ways of treating it is steam inhalation to help drainage. You can either do this by breathing, the vapour being given off by plain hot – not boiling – water, or you can add decongestant capsules containing natural essential oils, such as pine or eucalyptus. Inhaling this helps give relief from catarrh, nasal congestion and sinus trouble and can loosen mucus. Do not let the vapour come into contact with the eyes. You can also sprinkle the oils on to a handkerchief or tissue and breathe in the vapours that way.

Oxymetazoline hydrochloride drops can be prescribed. It's a vasoconstrictor – a drug that causes narrowing of the walls of blood vessels to relieve congestion. But it's usually inadvisable to use nose drops for longer than seven days, as they can cause a 'rebound' swelling and damage to the nasal passages, making matters worse.

If your symptoms become more severe and the sinuses are infected, the condition is then called sinusitis. Anyone who has ever suffered from this will remember all too well the typical throbbing headache which is made worse by bending over or blowing the nose. It's estimated that one in 200 colds leads to sinusitis.

The bones of the cheeks, forehead and back of the nose contain a hidden network of small caverns and channels – the sinuses – which help to make the bones lighter and give resonance to our voice. The mucus-secreting membrane that lines the nose continues on to form an interconnecting lining for all the sinuses. Normally there is free movement and circulation of air into and from the nose and sinuses. Likewise, mucus can drain from the sinuses. When germs or particles of dirt are inhaled, they lodge in the mucus; minute, moving 'hairs' called cilia then waft them to the back of the nose where they are harmlessly swallowed (the stomach's secretions are highly acidic and instantly destroy most germs) or are blown out on to a handkerchief.

However, if the lining membrane of the sinuses becomes inflamed – which is quite common after a heavy cold – more mucus than usual is produced, the cilia cease to function properly, infected secretions build up, the tiny drainage holes may become blocked and acute sinusitis results. The pain can be similar to that caused by toothache and the affected sinus – along the cheekbone below the eye, or just above the eyebrow, for example – may be tender to the touch. The sufferer will probably feel generally unwell and have a nasty headache and a blocked nose. He or she may also have a temperature and greeny discharge from the nose or running down the back of the throat.

An allergy – to irritant fumes or smoking, for instance – can also cause the lining membrane of the sinuses to swell and lead to a recurrent form of sinusitis. Diving and underwater swimming may have the same effect, if water is forced up into the sinuses.

An acute attack of sinusitis can usually be successfully treated by rest, painkillers and steam inhalations three times a day to relieve the congestion and help the sinuses to drain.

For a severe attack of sinusitis, your doctor may also prescribe antibiotics such as Amoxil or Erythromycin and, if symptoms do not improve or attacks recur, referral to a specialist may be necessary. Treatment may then include washing out the infected sinus under a local or general anaesthetic and finally an operation to improve the drainage system from the sinuses.

A constant and comfortable room temperature and a humid atmosphere (keep bowls of water by the radiators) should help, too. Some people also swear by an age-old remedy for catarrh and sinus trouble – garlic, in the form of garlic oil capsules, available from most chemists and health food shops.

Preparations prescribed Alevaire, ammonium chloride mixture, benzoin tinct., codeine linctus, diamorphine linctus, dihydrocodeine elixir, ephedrine nasal drops, Galcodine linctus, Galenphol linctus, isoaminile linctus, methadone linctus, menthol and eucalyptus inhalation, Pavacol-D, pholcodine linctus, simple linctus, Sudafed, xylometazoline nasal drops.

COLD SORES

Cold sores appear as little blisters which develop into weeping sores. They usually appear in groups around the lips but may also occur on other parts of the face. If precautions are not taken, the virus responsible can also be spread to other people, or to other parts of the body – the eye, for example – with potentially more serious results.

Cold sores are caused by the herpes simplex Type I virus, one of the herpes group of viruses, others of which cause chickenpox, shingles and glandular fever. A slightly different strain of the same virus, known as type II, is the one usually responsible for outbreaks of herpes blisters around the genital area, although type I may be the culprit here, too.

The herpes simplex type I virus is very common indeed – it's being passed around most of the time – and is responsible for many, if not most, sore throats, for example. This is one reason doctors would rather not prescribe antibiotics for uncomplicated sore throats; they know that antibiotics are not effective against viruses.

When they do prescribe antibiotics for a sore throat, they will do so to prevent those sore and inflamed throat tissues becoming infected by a secondary invasion of bacterial germs.

After the first infection, the herpes virus can lie dormant, causing no symptoms, in the nerve cells of the affected area. Under certain conditions, however, they may be reactivated and track up the same nerves to the same area of skin to produce further outbreaks of blisters.

Once the HSVI virus has entered the body, usually via the throat, it is carried around the body in the bloodstream and frequently establishes itself in a certain part of a nerve near the throat.

It rests there until our defences are lowered by a cold, for example, when it breaks out, travelling down the nerve to the lip or nose and causing an infection – the cold sore – on the surface. But it also inflames the nerve itself.

This nerve carries sensations from the area of the cold sore to the brain. It is 'overheated' by the virus and is felt as pain.

It is estimated that about half the adults in this country are carriers of type I herpes. Most of them will have had their first, often symptomless and undetected infection in early childhood. Many will never have another attack, some may have one after an interval of several years and a small percentage will have recurrent episodes every few months.

Various factors can contribute to reactivating the virus – exposure to sunlight, some infections and being generally 'run down' are amongst them. For a woman, an outbreak of cold sores is more likely during menstruation. However, with each new outbreak, the body produces further antibodies which accumulate to fight the virus. This means that, in time, outbreaks tend to lessen in both frequency and severity.

But for those severe outbreaks there are drugs available which are effective – the anti-viral drugs acyclovir (Zovirax) and idoxuridine (Herpid, Virudox). Treatment with Zovirax should be started as early as possible after the start of an infection. The cream should be applied five times a day at four-hourly intervals (don't worry about during the night). Carry on for five days. If healing isn't complete by that time, continue for another five days. Idoxuridine treatment should also be started as soon as possible – four times a day for four days. These products can sting when first applied.

Cold sores are highly contagious while the blisters are present. The virus is also found in the saliva of the sufferer and can be spread to others – so keep your kisses until the blisters have gone.

You can infect vulnerable parts of your own body, via the fingers, if you touch the sores and do not wash your hands afterwards. Any area of broken skin is especially susceptible. It is particularly important to avoid touching the blisters and then rubbing the eyes, as the virus may be transferred and cause an ulcer on the delicate membrane covering the eye. If this is not diagnosed and treated soon enough, it can damage the sight.

Mothers with cold sores should take extra care and wash their hands frequently, and always after applying medication. Babies and toddlers are extremely vulnerable to cold sores as they won't have had time to build up their antibodies. It is also important to keep the flannels, towels, eating and drinking utensils of the sufferer separate from those of the rest of the family.

With both types of herpes, close physical contact is needed before others are infected, so if reasonable precautions are taken during the week or so that the blisters last, there should be little cause for concern. The virus cannot be passed on while it is dormant and producing no symptoms but whenever you're infectious it is essential to protect others.

Many sufferers from recurrent cold sore notice definite warning symptoms before an outbreak – a 'prickly' feeling in the area of skin usually affected, for instance. If you apply the antiviral ointment or solution prescribed by your doctor during this phase, you can shorten the duration of the outbreak considerably. Cold-sore creams from the pharmacist can also help.

A simple old wives' remedy is to apply fresh, cold coffee to the area on a piece of clean cotton-wool every two or three hours and allow it to dry. It may sound primitive, but it appears to work for many people, so it is worth trying if a doctor or pharmacist isn't available. Other than this, the sores should just be kept clean and dry.

A regular, well-balanced diet will help maintain your general health and may therefore prevent attacks. So too may a good sun-blocking cream applied liberally to the lips before and during a concentrated period of sunbathing. But there is no cure for cold sores and if you are prone to them, keep a supply of cream in your medicine cupboard so that you can start the treatment when the warning symptoms first occur. Eventually you will develop your own natural resistance and cold sores should then become a thing of the past.

Preparations prescribed Herpid, Zovirax, Virudox

COLIC

Colic in babies is caused by bubbles of gas or air which become trapped in the immature digestive system. The consequent pain makes the baby cry, often inconsolably, and draw his or her legs up in pain. Problems with colic often appear when the baby is about three weeks old. They can be very wearing for the parents as well as the child, but don't despair, they usually stop of their own accord at about three months.

There are ways you can help soothe your colicky baby. Rocking or cuddling should help, and a car journey or pram ride will often send the baby off to sleep. Giving the age-old but new-formulated alcohol-free remedy, gripe water, has soothed many a baby's mother and sometimes the baby too!

Always ask your health visitor or doctor for advice the first time your baby screams inconsolably. The baby may be prescribed a medicine such as Infant Gaviscon. This contains sodium alginate, magnesium alginate and dried aluminium hydroxide. It reacts with gastric acid to form a viscous gel which, when mixed with stomach contents, thickens them and helps prevent reflux into the oesophagus. Infacol is a sugar-free, alcohol-free and colorant-free liquid to help relieve infant colic and griping pain. It contains activated dimethicone, which helps trap gas bubbles which the baby can bring up easily.

Infacol has a build-up effect which means it should be given for several days to achieve the best results.

Preparations prescribed Infacol, Infant Gavison

COLITIS AND CROHN'S DISEASE

Ulcerative colitis, an inflammation of the colon, affects the large bowel. Crohn's disease largely affects, or inflames, the small intestine. They used to be seen as two separate conditions, but they are both inflammatory diseases of the alimentary canal – the long tube which stretches from the mouth right down to the anus. It's not an exaggeration to say that inflammatory bowel disease can affect any part of the system because sometimes, though rarely, it is found in both the upper and lower sections – especially in Crohn's disease.

Although specialists still diagnose the two conditions separately, their management and treatment are quite similar in many respects. If surgery is required, however, the nature of the operation will depend on the location and extent of the inflammation.

If the disease is extensive or severe, the sufferers may need to go to the loo as many as twenty times a day. Yet some sufferers may not experience much more than a little diarrhoea, perhaps stained with blood or mucus, and some occasional abdominal pain. Others may not realise anything is wrong until they need an emergency operation for acute abdominal pain, where the inflammation has blocked the passage of food. The disease is unpredictable and will usually follow a course of waxing and waning.

Nowadays, much more is being done, both medically and socially to help sufferers. Thanks to the pioneering work of the National Association for Colitis and Crohn's disease (NACC), many sufferers who previously felt isolated and alone now realise that theirs is not an uncommon condition, that it can be managed and that it's nothing to be ashamed of.

The cause, however, is still not known. It could be that sufferers have an abnormal immune response in the colon, or that some kind of infection is the culprit. Contrary to popular opinion, the disease is not caused by stress or emotional upset – emotional upsets are usually a result of the disease. That's not to say that worry or a flu-type infection does not trigger an attack – this is highly likely. It's thought, too, that bowel infections, colds and even taking antibiotics or perhaps pain-killing drugs, could set off an attack.

Better drugs are available now for colitis sufferers, and surgical techniques have also progressed so that if an operation is needed, it can be designed to suit the individual's case history.

Sulphur drugs which help prevent flare-ups, and corticosteroids which damp down the inflammation (see STEROIDS, page 149) are the main drug treatments for ulcerative colitis. By damping down inflammation they help allow damaged tissue to heal.

Sulphasalazine (Salazopyrin) can be prescribed as tablets, enemas, suppositories and a suspension for the treatment of ulcerative colitis and Crohn's disease. It can cause unpleasant side-effects and blood, kidneys and your liver will need to be monitored for signs of toxicity. Sulphasalazine (particulary with higher doses) can cause nausea, vomiting, loss of appetite, ringing in the ears, headache and joint pain. The drug may colour the urine yellow.

For ulcerative colitis, mesalazine (Asacol, Pentasa, Salofalk) can be prescribed. It's one of the two components of sulphasalazine – the other being sulphapyridine. It's the latter which is said to be responsible for the majority of side-effects associated with sulphasalazine therapy while it is claimed that mesalazine is the active ingredient and, taken alone, causes fewer side-effects. Most common side-effects include gastrointestinal disturbances, headache and abdominal pain.

For local treatment of ulcerative colitis, ready-to-use, single-dose enemas or foam containing the corticosteroid, prednisolone (Predenema, Predfoam) can be prescribed. Administration of prednisolone via this route is seldom associated with adverse effects. Tablets containing the corticosteroid dexamethasone (Decadron) can be useful in ulcerative colitis.

Preparations prescribed Asacol, Colifoam, Decadron, Medrone, Merbentyl Syrup, Tablets, Pentasa, Precortisyl, Predenema, Predfoam, Prednesol, Salazopyrin

CONJUNCTIVITIS AND OTHER EYE INFECTIONS

Many of us will know what it's like to wake up in the morning with itchy, 'gritty'-feeling eyes and perhaps the eyelids stuck together. Underneath, the eyelids will be red and inflamed and the whites of the eyes probably bloodshot. Blinking may be painful and bright light distressing.

Conjunctivitis, as this condition is called, is very common and children are particularly prone to it. The symptoms are due to an inflammation of the conjunctiva – the delicate membrane that covers the whites of the eyes and the inner surfaces of the upper and lower eyelids. Where the membrane turns back on itself to cover both surfaces of the lids, sacs are formed, and small particles may collect here and irritate the conjunctiva – one cause of conjunctivitis.

Another possible cause is a viral or bacterial infection. Alternatively, the inflammation may be brought on by an allergic reaction – to pollens, animals hairs, cosmetics or the cleaning lotions used for contact lenses, for example.

It's perhaps surprising that conjunctivitis is not even more common than it is, since the eye is constantly exposed to various irritants and germs. Fortunately, the conjunctival sac is not an ideal breeding ground for germs, partly because of the cleansing effect of tear fluid. If a tear duct is blocked, then inflammation commonly develops and the duct will probably have to be unblocked. If, as well as being red and sore, the eyes are gummed up with sticky discharge – including perhaps some yellow pus – this usually means that the conjunctivitis is due to a virus or bacteria. This discharge will be particularly noticeable first thing in the morning, having accumulated during the night. The sufferer may also have a cold or other infection, such as, in the case of a child, measles. The discharge from the eyes is contagious, so keep handkerchiefs, towels, flannels and pillow cases separate to avoid spreading the germs to others. Your doctor will probably prescribe antibiotic eye drops and/or ointment to apply several times a day. Be sure to wash your hands both before and after doing so. The condition should improve within about four days – if not, referral to an eye specialist may be advised.

Another condition which causes irritating, sticky eyes is blepharitis, which I discuss later (see DANDRUFF, page 56). This is also treated by antibiotic eye drops or ointments.

Antibiotic ointments such as Genticin, which contains gentamicin (also useful for blepharitis) may also be needed for another infection of the eyelid at the root of the eyelashes, a stye. A stye is a small boil which instead of being in the hair root on the body like other boils, happens to be in the hair root of an eyelash. A more virulent germ than usual manages to 'crawl' down into the eyelash root and start it off. Corneal ulcers (ulcers on the front of the eye) also usually respond to the same type of treatment.

Conjunctivitis due to an allergy such as hay fever will usually produce a watery discharge and can often be relieved by special preventive eye drops such as Opticrom which contain sodium cromoglycate. This inhibits the release from hay-fever sensitised cells in the local tissues called mast cells of adrenalin-like chemicals which actually cause the symptoms. Wearing dark glasses can also help.

Sometimes town-dwellers will suffer from a persistent type of mild though distressing blepharitis/conjunctivitis known as 'urban eye', caused by irritant fumes and dust. Bathing the eyelids twice a day with a solution of one teaspoonful of bicarbonate of soda dissolved in one pint of recently boiled and cooled water can relieve the symptoms. Use a separate piece of cotton wool for each eye, bathing the edges of the closed lids, working inwards towards the nose.

It's best to avoid eye make-up during any attack of conjunctivitis – in fact it's possible that make-up is the cause. Likewise, if you wear contact lenses, revert to your spectacles while your eyes are inflamed and ask your doctor's or ophthalmic optician's advice on future use. And if your eyes become painful or your vision is affected, always consult your doctor without delay. These symptoms could indicate that there was inflammation within the eye and in that case urgent examination and treatment, probably by a specialist, would be required without delay.

Preparations prescribed Alomide, Chloromycetin Opthalmic Preparations, Cidomycin, Genticin, Minims Chloramphenicol, Minims Gentamicin Sulphate, Minims Neomycin Sulphate, Neo-Cortef, Neosporin, Noroxin, Opticrom, Periactin, Polyfax, Polytrim, Sno Phenicol, Sofradex, Soframycin

CONSTIPATION

Constipation in healthy people is a problem that's almost entirely preventable. Many people believe that eating a bit of extra fruit will soon cure constipation (medically speaking, being constipated usually means passing hard, pellet-like stools with considerable effort and straining), but this is unlikely to be enough. Bran, the outer husk of cereals, is the richest source of undigestible fibre. Wheat bran is the richest source of all. It's easy to increase your intake of bran by simply eating more wholemeal bread, flour and pastas, bran breakfast cereals, or sprinkling bran onto food. Also make sure you eat plenty of high fibre foods such as porridge oats, brown rice, baked beans, peas, lentils and sweetcorn, as well as plenty of fresh fruit and vegetables.

Remember that putting off going to the loo can lead to a loss of your usual bowel reflexes, which in turn causes constipation. Because of the straining associated with it, chronic constipation can lead to other unpleasant conditions such as piles, hiatus hernia and diverticuli – small 'blows outs' in the lining of the bowel which, if they become inflamed, develop into painful diverticulitis.

If you feel you do need a laxative there are many you can buy in the chemist or your doctor may prescribe you one. Laxatives go to work on the large intestine either by speeding up the progress of faecal matter passing through the bowel or by increasing its bulk. Stimulant laxatives such as senna make the bowel muscle contract to hurry the faeces along and bulk-forming laxatives such as ispaghula soak up water in the bowel to increase volume and make stools softer. Another is methylcellulose (Celevac) which absorbs water to swell to a soft gel of uniform consistency.

The laxatives phenolphthalein is often referred to as a stimulant laxative. What happens is this. As food passes down the alimentary canal, the stomach and small intestines require water in order to digest it. At this stage, the contents of the alimentary tract are fluid. There is a water conservation mechanism in the colon, where excess water is re-absorbed into the body, and this can cause constipation. The stimulant effect of phenolphthalein is that it stimulates the onward squeezing movements of the colon, which hampers water absorption because the bulk within the colon is moved on too quickly.

Other laxatives contain liquid paraffin, a lubricant which makes the faeces softer and easier to pass. Lactulose solution may be prescribed. This prevents the formation of hard stools and encourages normal bowel movement.

If you often find yourself resorting to laxatives, first check with your doctor that there is no underlying medical cause for your constipation – an underfunctioning thyroid gland is one possibility.

Preparations prescribed Bisacodyl, Carbalax, Celevac, co-danthramer suspension, co-danthrusate, Dioctyl, Fybogel, lactitol, lactulose solution, Manevac, Normacol, senna, sodium picosulphate, Trifyba

COUGHS

A cough is not an illness in itself, but a symptom. Although it can be irritating and often embarrassing, it is the body's natural response to any foreign body, congestion or irritation in the lungs or throat. The irritation may be due to things like air pollution or cigarette smoke, but in a great many cases it turns out to be the result of a cold or flu virus.

Sometimes, however, coughing signals a more serious disorder in the respiratory tract, so it is extremely important to seek medical advice for any cough that lasts for longer than a few days or if there are streaks of blood in any mucus you cough up.

Coughing up green sputum probably signifies a bacterial infection which may need antibiotics.

Coughs can be treated with cough suppressants or expectorants. Cough suppressants, as the name suggests, are medicines that suppress the symptom, the cough itself, without tackling the underlying cause. They reduce the frequency and intensity of a cough by acting on the part of the brain that controls the coughing reflex, or at the site of irritation in the throat. These may help if you have a dry hacking cough. Dry coughs occur when there is irritation but little phlegm in the larynx at the top of the windpipe, or in the pharynx, the cavern between the mouth and nose at the top and the oesophagus (gullet) and trachea (windpipe) below. This irritation stimulates the cough reflex, the body's natural response. Pholcodine exerts an inhibitory action on the cough centre and has a less constipating effect than codeine, for example.

Expectorants relieve chesty coughs, the type you often get as a result of a cold or flu. These medicines claim to loosen the 'debris' or phlegm in order to make it easier to cough up.

Some cough medicines can cause drowsiness. If a medicine makes you drowsy do not drive or operate machinery. And avoid alcoholic drink. Children being given cough medicines which may cause drowsiness should not be left on their own.

If you do have an irritating cough and want something to relieve it, describe your cough to your pharmacist and take his or her advice. You don't want to buy something that may make your cough worse. As always, you should tell your pharmacist if you are taking any other medication, have a medical condition or are pregnant or think you may be.

Despite the enormous number of cough remedies available, there is disagreement as to their value. They may give temporary relief to a tickly throat and taste pleasant, even soothing, but they may not be any more effective than a honey drink you have made yourself or inhaling steam to ease congestion. Doctors are sometimes reluctant to prescribe cough suppressants because coughing is a protective reflex; repeated bouts of coughing can be distressing, however, so soothing medication may be needed.

When patients are well in themselves but the troublesome cough is keeping them awake at night and to no good purpose, then I'm in favour of cough suppressants.

See COLD, THE COMMON, page 37, for preparations prescribed.

CRADLE CAP

Cradle cap is a harmless condition resembling dandruff that is extremely common in young babies. It usually appears during the first three months of a baby's life, but can also affect toddlers and young children. If your baby develops cradle cap, you may first of all notice a little scurf on his or her head, followed by the appearance of yellowish or brownish greasy-looking scales of thickened skin which stick to the scalp. These patches sometimes appear over the whole head, sometimes just in small areas. Some specialists believe the crusts are due to excess production of sebum – grease from the sebaceous glands – in response to the mother's hormones.

Although it can be unsightly, cradle cap is unlikely to do your baby any harm. It usually disappears on its own after a few months. To ease it you can rub the baby's head with baby oil or olive oil and leave for 24 hours. Comb the hair gently, then wash the flakes of skin away. Alternatively, treat cradle cap with specially formulated gentle, medicated shampoo available from the chemist. If you are worried and the cradle cap persists seek the advice of your doctor who may prescribe a shampoo such as Capasal which contains salicylic acid, coconut oil and distilled coal tar. This will help loosen the flakes and moisturise the scalp.

Preparations prescribed Capasal

CUTS AND GRAZES

You can treat most cuts and grazes at home quite safely, but always wash your hands first, if possible. Clean the cut by holding it under running water, or by gently wiping it with an antiseptic wipe or cotton wool soaked in warm water. It's best to use a fresh piece of cotton wool for each wipe. Some small cuts will still bleed quite profusely at first, so if this is happening after a few minutes, you'll need to apply pressure to stem the flow. Press a pad, a clean tissue for example, firmly over the cut for a few minutes.

If you like to use plasters and antiseptic ointments on cuts and grazes, fine – it will do no harm. Personally, I prefer not to use ointments and I use plasters mainly to keep dirt out of the wound. When that isn't necessary or the injury is small, it will heal up nicely if left alone. If a cut is very large or deep, if it has rugged or gaping edges, if something is embedded in it or if it is a deep cut with only a small opening in the skin (this might happen if the culprit is a rusty nail, for example) always seek medical help – you may need an injection to up-date your tetanus protection with such wounds. For secondary infections of cuts, grazes and wounds you may need an antibiotic ointment.

Preparations prescribed Cetavlex, Genticin, Polyfax

CYSTITIS

Cystitis is a subject that regularly fills my postbag – hardly surprising when you realise that it's one of the most common complaints suffered by women (men and children can be affected too). It's also likely that more than half the women in the UK contract it at some time. Cystitis is an inflammation of the bladder lining and the urethra – the tube down which urine is excreted from the bladder. The most common symptoms are a frequent need to pass urine, accompanied by a burning sensation and pain around the pubic bone low down in the front.

Some women experience attacks several times a year and an unfortunate few are seldom free of the problem. That's because a woman's anatomy makes her particularly prone to cystitis. Unlike a man's, her urethra is very short and the normally harmless germs around the anus are easily able to track upwards to the bladder, whose natural defences may be unable to cope with them.

Inflammation then develops and often spreads to the urethra – a condition known as urethritis – which results in the typical burning pain as urine is passed. The urine is often dark brown and strong smelling; it may also contain traces of blood, so don't be alarmed if this happens to you. The sufferer has a constant urge to 'spend a penny' even though there is little or nothing to pass. A slight temperature, nausea, a dragging feeling in the lower abdomen and tenderness over the bladder are also common, as is a general feeling of being unwell.

Don't be misled into thinking that if you have cystitis you must necessarily have an infection. The delicate lining of the urethra and/or the bladder can, in those susceptible, react to irritants such as scented soap, powders, vaginal deodorants, bath oils and the detergents used to wash clothes. Some people are sensitive to highly spiced foods, strong tea, coffee, alcohol and fruit juices. Friction or bruising during lovemaking can also inflame the tissues, as the urethra is just above the vaginal entrance – a lubricant jelly may then help by overcoming any dryness. Hormone replacement therapy or oestrogen cream may be more effective after the menopause.

Germs can also be inadvertently 'helped' into the urethra during intercourse. Inserting tampons can do this too, as can wiping yourself from back to front (instead of front to back) after a bowel movement. The main germ which causes trouble here and after sexual intercourse is one called *Escherichia coliform,* more commonly known as *E. coli.* It lives in the bowel, where it is harmless, but if it makes its way to the vagina or urethra it can cause problems.

Thrush infection, perhaps aggravated by wearing tight-fitting trousers, is another possible cause of symptoms. It is important, too, to pass urine as soon as you feel the need and to empty your bladder completely each time by squeezing out every last drop – a reservoir of urine can make a fertile breeding ground for germs.

So, if you are prone to cystitis, always wash around your vaginal area and 'spend a penny' both before and after making love. Having sex with a full bladder, or bowel for that matter, means bruising is more likely to occur, which can also encourage cystitis. Ask your partner to wash daily, too. Try to drink at least three or four pints of water every day to flush out any germs and keep the urine dilute and so less irritant.

If symptoms do develop, neutralising the acidity is a

worthwhile first line of treatment, since as many as two out of three sufferers won't actually have any infection and the symptoms should therefore settle in a day or so using this method alone. Start immediately symptoms appear by drinking a pint of water with a teaspoonful of bicarbonate of soda added – unless you suffer from high blood pressure, or heart or kidney trouble, in which case consult your doctor first. Drink a pint of this mixture every hour for three hours, interspersed with other soft drinks. This will change the urine from acid to alkaline and relieve the pain, but bicarbonate of soda, especially in a sufferer whose kidneys are not working properly, could lead to side-effects such as a rise in blood pressure.

Alternatively, and better and safer, you could take potassium citrate or a specially formulated, pleasant-tasting medicine from the chemist. These medicines mainly contain sodium citrate which makes the urine less acid, and are usually meant to be taken regularly for 48 hours. Such treatments can be very helpful, but if symptoms persist after the 48 hours are up, you should see your doctor – take a specimen of urine with you in a clean, screw-topped jar. As I've said in as many as two thirds of cases of cystitis, there's no infection. But the remainder will usually need to be prescribed antibiotics to cure any infection. There are many antibiotics used in the treatment of urinary tract infections. These include ampicillin, amoxycyllin and pivampicillin, trimethoprim, and nitrofurantoin.

If your symptoms come back regularly, see your doctor for advice.

Preparations prescribed Cymalon, Hiprex, MacroBID, Macrodantin, Mictral, Utinor

DANDRUFF AND SEBORRHOEIC DERMATITIS

Dandruff is a condition rather like acne which, although not serious, can be acutely embarrassing to those who suffer from it and a source of amusement to those who don't. It is also the most common cause of itching of the scalp, but is not a sign of general ill health.

Normally, everyone's skin cells, including those in their scalp, are replenished about every 28 days and the top layer is regularly shed in minute, usually unnoticeable pieces. In dandruff sufferers, this process may be speeded up and the particles shed are larger and easily seen. With milder forms of dandruff, sometimes known as scurf, the flakes of skin are dry and white and tend to clump together in the hair. Touching the hair – which most people do many times a day without realising it – dislodges the fragments and they fall on to the shoulders, looking like a white powder.

This type of dandruff can usually be controlled by washing the hair two or three times a week with a medicated, anti-dandruff shampoo. These often contain tar, sulphur or salicylic acid to soften and help loosen scale and scalp debris. Other anti-dandruff shampoos for more severe cases contain selenium sulphide to reduce the development of dandruff by slowing down the growth of skin cells, as well as having mild antifungal properties. Antibacterial gels, such as Capitol, which contain benzalkonium chloride may be useful.

There is, however, a more severe form of dandruff called seborrhoeic dermatitis of the scalp, which may not respond to these shampoos. It can occur on other parts of the body, too, and may be very difficult to treat effectively.

Seborrhoeic dermatitis can affect both children and adults. On a baby's scalp it is known as cradle cap and the condition often also appear as a nappy rash for which your doctor can prescribe a cream. For adults and older children, Capasal Therapeutic Shampoo may help, as it 'dissolves' the skin flakes but also contains a moisturiser to protect the skin from dehydration. Efalith ointment, containing lithium succinate and zinc sulphate, can be applied twice daily in the morning and evening. This dosage regime should be continued until improvement occurs, usually within four weeks. It may then be possible to keep up this improvement by applying the ointment now and again. Severe dandruff or psoriasis of the scalp may also respond to a scalp lotion containing a topical steroid such as fluocinonide (Metosyn).

It used to be thought that when they occurred in adults, both seborrhoeic dermatitis and other forms of dandruff were due to over-production of sebum. Diet, hygiene, climate and stress were also thought to play a part. However, recent research has shown that it is the sufferer's over-reaction to a minute, fungus-like organism called *Pityrosporum ovale*. It is the reaction to the fungus, rather than the fungus itself, that causes the scalp's top layer of skin to flake off as dandruff, or gives rise to the symptoms of seborrhoeic dermatitis.

In this condition, which is most common in young men but can affect women, too, the flakes of skin are large, yellow and oily. The skin on the scalp becomes red, inflamed and soggy, especially around the edges and may be infected by other germs. Eyelashes, eyebrows, skin folds on either side of the nose and behind the ears can all be affected, as can other parts of the body, such as the chest, armpits, breasts and groin.

Neither dandruff nor seborrhoeic dermatitis is catching, because, as I said, it is not the fungus itself that produces the symptoms – as it is with athlete's foot, for instance – but an over-reaction to it which only occurs in susceptible people. The fungus itself is around all the time. Why some people and not others have this susceptibility isn't known.

If you find your dandruff cannot be controlled by medicated shampoos, there are more effective treatments your doctor can prescribe. The same advice applies if you think you have seborrhoeic dermatitis. Your doctor's examination will exclude other possible skin conditions such as psoriasis and eczema, and suitable treatment can then be suggested.

If dandruff or scalp symptoms are severe, there is now some good news for sufferers. A specific antifungal shampoo called Nizoral is available on prescription and is very effective. Your doctor may suggest using this twice weekly for about four weeks, interspersed with milder medicated shampoos on other days. You may then be advised to use the antifungal shampoo less frequently to prevent symptoms recurring, once every one to two weeks perhaps. Regular hair-washing with this shampoo may also help if your eyelids are inflamed and crusty, although another organism – the staphylococcus – is often involved in this case too. It causes a condition known as blepharitis, to which many people are prone from childhood. Symptoms can usually be controlled by removing crusts from the eyelids by bathing them with a cotton wool bud dipped in baby shampoo, diluted to half strength, and then applying an antibiotic ointment to the rims.

Your doctor may prescribe antifungal and/or various anti-inflammatory applications for skin rashes on other parts of the body due to seborrhoeic dermatitis; taking an antibiotic by mouth may be necessary if the rash becomes infected by other germs. A general one may be used unless the doctor takes a swab to find out which germs are present and so prescribe a specific antibiotic to counteract that germ. So, if the usual medicated shampoos do not keep your dandruff at bay, don't feel that it is too minor a problem to bother your doctor with. Any of these conditions can be very distressing and embarrassing and there is a lot that can now be done to treat them.

Preparations prescribed Balneum with Tar, Baltar-Shampoo, Capasal, Capitol, Efalith, Elocon, Ionil, Locoid Scalp Lotion, Metosyn, Nizoral, Pragmatar, Synalar range

DEPRESSION

Depression is a common medical condition, often described as a continuing feeling of despondency, despair and sadness. It affects around one in four women and one in ten men at some time in their lives. Symptoms can also include sleep disturbances, lethargy and difficulty in concentrating and sudden mood swings. Sex drive and appetite can be affected, too.

Depression can vary enormously in its severity and in the form it takes, producing different symptoms in different people. Some people stop sleeping while others can't get enough sleep. Some become hyperactive, particularly those with manic depression, while at the other extreme some people just sit, in a seemingly frozen state, without facial expression or any desire to move.

It can be a difficult condition for a person to come to terms with – especially when friends and family who do not realise that it is a medical condition may not be particularly sympathetic and believe the sufferer should just 'snap out of it'. It can be difficult, too, for doctors to treat people with depression. Triggers for depression can include a bereavement, divorce, retirement, redundancy, serious illness or injury, or just loneliness.

Although it's also thought that depression could be caused by a lack of certain chemical messengers in the brain, no one treatment is necessarily right so it becomes a matter of trial and error.

'Major' tranquillisers, those usually only prescribed by psychiatrists (see ANXIETY page 20) and anti-depressant drugs, are one of the most important and vital parts of that treatment. If the depression has become so severe and the person has to be admitted to hospital, then electroconvulsive therapy becomes another alternative. But ECT suffers from bad publicity. It's been portrayed as something barbaric and terrible, and certainly in the early days it could be fairly awful. But not today. Most specialists would agree that for certain types of depression there is no alternative to ECT. Without it, some people with depression would take their own lives or at least would never recover. It is, literally, a shock treatment and can, just as an emotional shock, help them climb out of depression. For some people, the chance of successful treatment without ECT would be bleak to non-existent.

There are alternatives, such as counselling from a professional who is skilled and qualified. Talking to a person who is sympathetic and able to listen can achieve a cure by itself if the patient is able to unburden themselves and learn to understand why he or she is depressed. Feelings have to be worked through before any moves can be made towards re-establishing a happy and fulfilling life.

Do bear in mind that depression isn't always as straightforward as we assume it to be and the expected symptoms – black feelings and waking up in the middle of the night, for example – are not always dramatically present in everyone who is depressed. Depression can take many guises and a sensitive doctor will often be aware of an underlying depression following problems at work or some other setback. Your doctor may reach the conclusion that a short course of anti-depressant tablets is required to allow you to cope better with your life while you are sorting out any current problems. Or, a recently introduced medicine may be prescribed. Called Manerix (moclobemide), it's a new type of antidepressant. No special dietary restrictions are necessary when taking these tablets. But as some patients may be especially sensitive to tyramine you'll be advised not to eat large quantities of food containing it – mature cheese, yeast extracts and fermented soya bean products (contained in some Chinese foods). Some of the adverse effects of this new medicine include sleep disturbances, dizziness, feeling sick, headache, confusion.

Anti-depressants are useful and effective drugs for depression – even though it has to be said that, according to MIND, the National Association for Mental Health, for about three depressed people in every ten they have no useful effect whatsoever. And each year about 400 people use anti-depressant drugs as the means to end their lives. Yet anti-depressant drugs are the most common form of treatment for depression and they do enable many thousands of people to lead worthwhile lives.

There are many anti-depressants. The main groups are tricyclic anti-depressants – examples include amitriptyline, clomipramine hydrochloride, imipramine hydrochloride. These are usually the first type to be prescribed for someone who is depressed. They work by acting on chemical processes in the brain – effectively changing a person's sensitivity to emotions.

The other group is MAOIs – monoamine-oxidase inhibitor anti-depressants – usually prescribed when sufferers found no relief after taking one of the tricyclics. Examples are isocarboxazid and phenelzine. These drugs increase the levels of neurotransmitters by blocking the action of the enzyme that breaks them down. They can affect the way certain foods are digested and can cause them to become poisonous. Cheese, Bovril, Marmite, Oxo and other meat and yeast extracts should be avoided. Other food to be avoided include broad bean pods, pickled herrings, bananas, yoghurt, chocolate, canned figs and certain red wines and sherry.

Some drugs to treat depression combine an anti-depressant with a minor tranquilliser and an anti-depressant with a major tranquilliser.

Anti-depressants can cause a large number of side-effects. These include a dry mouth, sedation, blurred vision, constipation, feeling nauseous, passing water less often, lower blood pressure, changes in heart rhythm, sweating, trembling hands, rashes, disturbed behaviour, confusion, reduced sexual arousal, dizziness. And many people do experience withdrawal symptoms when they stop taking anti-depressants. Coming off anti-depressants is easier if the dose is reduced slowly.

Preparations prescribed Anafranil, Asendis, Camcolit, Concordin, Faverin, Gamanil, Lentizol, Limbitrol, Ludiomil, Manerix, Molipaxin, Nardil, Pertofran, Seroxat, Surmontil, Tofranil, Triptafen, Tryptizol, Vivalan

DIABETES

Diabetes affects about two per cent of the population. *Diabetes mellitus* is a condition in which the body can't properly use sugar and carbohydrates from the food eaten. It's insulin that enables body tissues to take up glucose from the blood. So the cause of diabetes is the failure of the pancreas to produce insulin, the reason why this happens is still being investigated. In children, viruses may play a part.

There are two types of diabetes – insulin-dependent diabetes and non-insulin dependent diabetes. The first (insulin-dependent) is treated by insulin injections and diet. About one in four people with diabetes have this type. It's the most severe form and usually develops under the age of 30.

Non-insulin dependent diabetes affects the remaining three out of four people with diabetes. It's also known as maturity-onset diabetes and is more common among elderly people, particularly those who are overweight. Certain drugs such as corticosteroids and diuretics, by altering the way the body deals with glucose, can trigger the signs of diabetes. So can an illness like pancreatitis.

What happens is that insulin is produced, but not in the amounts the body needs. Warning signs can include feeling very thirsty, eating and drinking more, tiredness and a frequent need to pass urine. Non-insulin dependent diabetes is treated by diet alone (a reduction in the consumption of sugary foods), or, for about half of the people with this form of diabetes, with drugs and diet. The drugs stimulate extra insulin production. They're called sulphonylurea drugs – examples are glibenclamide; chlorpropamide and tolbutamide (in conjunction with diet). Side-effects of these drugs include dizziness, confusion, weakness and sweating.

Guar gum is also used to help treat diabetes. It's used to slow the rate of glucose absorption, thereby reducing the after-meal peak in the blood-glucose level. This may allow a reduction in dosage of insulin or oral hypoglycaemic agents – which won't have so much work to do since the sugars are not being absorbed so quickly into the blood stream.

All forms of diabetes need proper medical treatment. Without it the disease can be life-threatening, by causing a hyperglycaemic coma. Treatment should also help to control the other known complications such as blindness, heart disease, kidney damage and gangrene.

Losing weight and taking more exercise may be all that's needed for some people to control their non-insulin dependent diabetes.

Preparations prescribed Daonil, Euglucon, Glurenorm, Guarina, Rastinon

DIARRHOEA

Diarrhoea involves loose or liquid bowel movements and frequent or speedy trips to the loo. It is also often accompanied by cramping pain in the lower abdomen. Most attacks are caused by gastro-intestinal infections – you can think of them as the body's way of getting rid of harmful substances. If more than one member of your family suffers at the same time, it is likely the diarrhoea was caused by something you've all eaten. If you have just come back from a trip away, you might have been exposed to standards of hygiene that do not match up to what you are used to, resulting in what we know as 'holiday tummy'. If your diarrhoea is accompanied by vomiting, food poisoning is also a likely cause. Gastric flu could be the culprit, too.

Another common cause of diarrhoea is stress. A job

interview or a driving test can reduce the toughest of us to a bundle of nerves. Eating large amounts of food with laxative properties, such as prunes, can have an adverse effect. Diarrhoea can be a side-effect of taking certain drugs – antibiotics, for example. Tetracycline, a commonly prescribed antibiotic, can destroy friendly bacteria which normally live in the bowel and are part of our natural defences against more harmful bacteria. If these are destroyed, the harmful ones – perhaps resistant to the antibiotics – can thrive. But if this happens to you, don't just stop taking the antibiotics. Ring your doctor and ask for advice.

Whatever the cause, most attacks of diarrhoea usually clear up quickly and without medical attention. The best way to treat yourself is by not eating for 24 hours and drinking plenty of water or well-diluted drinks. Frequent bursts of diarrhoea can make you feel even more ill as your body becomes dehydrated. The greatest risk from diarrhoea, and from vomiting too, is that the body's essential minerals are lost at the same time. Mineral depletion of this nature can make you feel weak and eventually faint. In a healthy person, water is essential to maintain normal body functions. Its importance is underlined by the fact that around half our body weight is water. Normally our kidneys balance the water lost in the urine and through perspiration against our fluid intake. For example, we pass less urine in hot weather because we can perspire several litres in a day. Consequently, our kidneys concentrate the wastes that we need to pass and conserve the body's water content for the temporarily more important work of keeping our temperature stable. Also, our thirst is stimulated so that we feel more thirsty and therefore drink more in hot weather.

Diarrhoea or sickness causes excessive loss of fluid, but if we are feeling ill, we may not feel thirsty. This means that our water balance is upset and we will continue to feel unwell until the fluid balance is restored.

To prevent mineral loss and dehydration you can buy ready-prepared sachets to be mixed with water, which are a combination of essential salts, minerals and energy-giving glucose. (This is known as oral rehydration therapy.) When these are mixed with the correct quantity of water as instructed, they are just the right strength for quick absorption, even by an inflamed stomach. They can also be prescribed by your doctor.

Medicines used to treat diarrhoea include powders which form a bulky mass inside the bowel to help carry away irritant substances. Typical examples are aluminium silicate (kaolin), calcium carbonate (chalk) and pectin (a purified carbohydrate product made from citrus fruits). Preparations made with these powders contain particles that swell up as they absorb water from the large intestine. This makes the faeces firmer and less runny. It's thought that these powders may absorb irritants and harmful chemicals along with the excess water.

Other drugs act on the muscular bowel wall to slow down bowel movements, relieving the familiar griping pains caused by diarrhoea. Typical examples are drugs from the opium family like codeine phosphate or morphine, which is usually mixed with kaolin, or a medicine such as Lomotil (diphenoxylate hydrochloride and atropine sulphate) which is an opiate and anticholinergic – and can cause allergic reactions, central nervous system upsets such as lethargy and restlessness among others; or the opiate Imodium (loperamide hydrochloride) – which can cause rashes.

In normally healthy adults, diarrhoea is rarely a serious condition. Children and the elderly may suffer much more. This is because they are more sensitive to the problems of dehydration and often have less body fluid to lose. Babies under six months old are at the greatest risk from dehydration. Their metabolic rate is high, their kidneys don't yet retain water very efficiently and they lose a greater proportion of water compared to their weight than adults do.

But even if you're a healthy adult, you should always consult your doctor if the condition doesn't improve within 48 hours, if the faeces contain blood, if there is severe abdominal pain or vomiting, or if you've just returned from a foreign country.

To help avoid gyppy tummy and the holiday runs – or worse – be especially careful about the ice in the long, cool drinks. And if the only available restaurant doesn't look too clean, stick to mass-produced bottled drinks and thoroughly cooked food.

Preparations prescribed Celevac, Dioralyte, Electrolade, Imodium, Lomotil, Rehidrat

DRY SKIN CONDITIONS – ECZEMA, DERMATITIS AND PSORIASIS

Eczema and dermatitis are used as virtually interchangeable terms and generally mean inflammation of the skin. The main symptoms are itching and redness, accompanied by small blisters which often weep and form a crust. Eczema can take the form of small red patches on the limbs or it can afflict large areas of the body. Although it is not usually a 'serious disease', nor a contagious one, it can be severe, uncomfortable and unsightly, causing the sufferer to become exceptionally self-conscious. If you think you have eczema, see your doctor. Although it is often hard to define the cause of eczema or to cure it completely, there are a number of treatments available to control it – emollients, antipruritics, topical steroids, antifungals and antibiotics.

You can help combat the dryness, itching and flaking by preserving the moisture content of your skin. Avoid harsh or highly perfumed soaps or bath additives; instead, try using emollient (moisturising) soaps, creams and specially made bath oils, and when bathing use warm water instead of hot. These emollient products can be helpful when the skin becomes generally dry – often one of the minor complaints of pregnancy. Moisturising bath oils can make the surface of the bath slippery, so do be careful about getting in and out.

Dry skin conditions can be a problem in childhood. About one child in ten suffers from infantile or atopic eczema. The symptoms are similar to those described above, but may look worse as a result of the child's scratching. Consult your doctor for treatment and advice. At home, keep the child's skin away from direct contact with wool or other rough fabrics – choose soft, pure cotton instead. Keep the child's fingernails short and use only gentle cleansing products suitable for infants.

Another form of skin complaint is known as contact dermatitis. This has similar symptoms to eczema but is specifically caused by contact with substances to which your skin is sensitive – household detergents or costume jewellery, for example. Protect your hands when using household cleansing fluids or chemicals, etc., and avoid contact with metals, dyes or even washing powders which may cause you problems. If you're not sure of the cause, consult your doctor, who may choose to carry out allergy tests. A mild hydrocortisone cream will ease discomfort by reducing inflammation and calming irritated skin. Hydrocortisone provides anti-inflammatory action yet is the least potent topical corticosteroid available.

Psoriasis can vary in severity from being a mild nuisance to, rarely, being so severe that the sufferer has to be admitted to hospital. With psoriasis, the skin cells grow much faster than usual. Normally, the skin cells divide and shed every 25 to 28 days. In cases of psoriasis this happens in just three to four days.

The precise cause isn't clear. There's evidence to suggest that it could be partly genetic and partly environmental. What is known is that psoriasis can be triggered by stress, some drugs (beta-blockers given for high blood pressure, for example) and even an infection with a virus, such as German measles. The most common form, plaque psoriasis, usually develops as scattered, raised red patches with thick, silvery white scales on the skin, usually on the knees, elbows and scalp. On the scalp it's most noticeable as a thick white encrustation around the hairline and ears.

Psoriasis seems to be linked to heredity and can appear at any age, though it most commonly attacks those in their teens or twenties, affecting men and women equally. It can be a difficult condition to treat and unfortunately there's no long-term cure. Outbreaks tend to come and go – frequency and extent vary between individuals and cannot be predicted accurately.

Although psoriasis is not often harmful to the general health and is not catching, the appearance of the skin can cause the sufferer great embarrassment and discomfort, especially when large areas are involved. The condition normally improves in the summer and gets worse again in the winter, but patches will sometimes clear up completely for years. On a day-to-day basis, emollient baths and creams (E45 for example) rubbed into the scaly patches can help to soothe the itching and flaking. Yoga, meditation and methods of relaxation – including holidays, especially in the sun, which is extremely beneficial for psoriasis – can all bring relief and, by encouraging a calmer outlook, may help prevent further flare-ups.

Sufferers can also benefit from eating more fish, especially oily fish like mackerel and herring. It's been suggested that one of the unsaturated fats in fish oils, EPA, is able to replace, within the body, another unsaturated fat, arachidonic acid. It is the metabolism – the body's usage – of this last acid which seems to be upset in someone who suffers from psoriasis.

But despite all these possible remedies, active outbreaks should always be seen by a doctor. If the psoriasis is widespread or persistent, specialised hospital treatments will be recommended.

Epogam contains a special variety of evening primrose oil. The major active constituent is gamolenic acid, also known as gamma-linolenic acid (GLA). It had been thought for some time that patients with atopic eczema may not be able to use dietary linoleic acid normally. So that it can perform its functions, this essential nutrient must be converted within the body to GLA. Research carried out by Scotia Pharmaceuticals showed that eczema sufferers fail to convert linoleic acid to GLA normally and do not make enough GLA for normal skin structure and function. Adding GLA to the diet can help correct this biochemical abnormality.

It's worth remembering that once the eczema improves the dosage may be reduced to a lower maintenance dose, but if treatment stops the patient's eczema may recur. According to the National Eczema Society, Epogam may take eight to 12 weeks to begin to be effective. The main benefit appears to be a reduction of the itch and a reduction in the need for steroids and antibiotics. So far no major adverse effects have been reported although nausea, indigestion and headache have occurred occasionally.

Topical steroids (see STEROIDS, page 149) are useful treatments in dry skin conditions such as eczema, dermatitis and psoriasis. They help reduce the redness and itchiness. These creams containing topical steroids such as hydrocortisone, clobetasone butyrate (Eumovate Ointment), beclomethasone dipropionate (Propaderm Ointment), or clobetasol propionate (Dermovate Cream). Sometimes infection can also be a problem in these skin conditions. When this is a problem, topical steroid cream with an antibacterial agent and/or a an antifungal agent can be effective, for example a cream such as Dermovate-NN Ointment which contains clobetasol propionate (a topical steroid), neomycin (an antibacterial agent) and nystatin (an anticandidal agent).

But excessive use of topical steroids can increase the risk of absorption through the skin and the risk of side-effects. Too much may result in thinning of the skin.

Dithranol, a synthetic chemical, is an effective topical

treatment for plaque psoriasis in hospitals. Newer creams and ointments containing it have become available (Psoradrate, Dithrocream, Dithrolan, Anthranol) so that treatment can be carried out at home. But it does stain the skin and will stain bedding and clothing. For this reason treated areas are usually covered by tubular gauze in an effort to keep the drug off clothing. It's irritant and if not used carefully will actually burn the skin. The staining of the skin is only superficial, and when the treatment is stopped the skin soon returns to normal.

For severe extensive psoriasis which seems to be resistant to other forms of therapy, a medicine such as Tigason (etretinate) may be prescribed. This is a vitamin A derivative. It could harm an unborn child, so women who may become pregnant shouldn't use this medicine and contraception should be used for at least a month before treatment, during treatment and for at least two years afterwards. Most frequent side-effects are dryness of the mouth and lips, itching, hair thinning and hair loss (alopecia) – which is reversible when treatment is stopped. Sometimes the levels of blood fats rise as a result of the drug, and this may be monitored by regular blood tests.

Preparations prescribed Alcoderm Cream/Lotion, Alphaderm Cream, Alphodith, Alphosyl, Alphosyl HC Cream, Anthranol, Aquadrate Cream, Balneum, Balneum Plus, Balneum with Tar, Baltar Shampoo, Betnovate Cream, Betnovate Ointment, Betnovate Lotion, Betnovate-N Ointment, Betnovate RD Ointment, Daktacort, Dermovate Cream, Dermovate-NN Ointment, Dermovate-NN Cream, Diprobase, Diprobath, Diprosalic, Diprosone, Dithrocream, Dithrolan, Efcortelan Cream or Ointment, Elocon, Epogam, Epogam Paediatric, Eumovate Ointment or Cream, Eurax Hydrocortisone, Gentisone HC Cream/Ointment, Gentisone HC Ear Drops, Hydrocal, Hydrocortisyl skin cream and ointment, Lipobase, Locoid C Cream or ointment, Locoid Lipocream, Metosyn Scalp Lotion, Metosyn FapG Cream, Metosyn Ointment, Mildison Lipocream, Modrasone, Neotigason, Nerisone Cream, Oily Cream and Ointment, Nerisone Forte Oily Cream and Ointment, Nutraplus Cream, Periactin, Preferid Cream/Ointment, Propaderm Ointment or Cream, Psoradrate Cream, Psorigel, Quin-cocort Cream, Soframycin, Sofra-tulle, Sudocrem, Synalar Range, Tarcortin, Tavegil, Tigason, Timodine, Topilar, TriAdcortyl, Tri-Cicatrin Ointment, Ultradil, Ultralanum, Unguentum Merck

EAR INFECTIONS

Otitis media is, more simply, a painful infection of the middle ear. It's the type of infection that young children are particularly prone to because their natural antibodies are not yet fully developed. Also, the eustacian tubes which connect the back of the nose are shorter and more horizontal than they will be in adulthood. Both of these factors allow germs to enter the middle ear more readily in childhood.

These infections are treated with paracetamol to reduce pain and also by the use of decongestants or antihistamines to reduce any swelling in the eustachian tube. This enables any pus to come out of the middle ear. Sometimes antibiotics are prescribed as a safeguard even though they do not combat viral infections, responsible for a high proportion of such infections. But when it comes to ear infections it's not always easy to establish whether or not the infection is viral or bacterial. The antibiotics used are, for example, ampicillin, amoxycillin and pivampicillin.

For inflammation of the outer ear, *otitis externa*, corticosteroid ear drops can be given when there's no infection, to reduce swelling. When there is infection, drops containing an antibiotic and a corticosteroid such as Gentisone HC Ear drops (gentamicin sulphate and hydrocortisone acetate) may be given, for the treatment of eczema and infection of the outer ear particularly as in such infections the offending organisms are often varied and difficult to identify. Antibiotic drops can be prescribed or sometimes antibiotics administered orally. Doctors prefer not to use antibiotics long-term since the skin may become sensitive to the antibiotic and become inflamed. The early antibiotics were the most notorious offenders. That is why penicillin is rarely, if ever, used in cream or drop form.

Both types of ear problem need medical attention because they can lead to deafness.

Preparations prescribed Audax, Cidomycin Ear Drops, Genticin Ear Drops, Gentisone HC Ear Drops, Klaricid Paediatric Suspension, Locorten-Vioform Ear Drops, Neo-Cortef Ear Drops or Ointment, Otomize Ear Spray, Otosporin, Sofradex Ear Drops and Ointment, Tri-Adcortyl

EAR WAX

Everyone has a certain amount of wax in their ears – it is a natural substance secreted by tiny glands in the skin of the ear similar to sweat glands. It helps protect the sensitive lining in the outer channel of the ear from infection and keeps it free of dust and flakes of skin. And just as some people sweat more than others, some people naturally produce more ear wax.

Usually the wax steadily crumbles away and is expelled from the ear as tiny flakes, to be replaced by a fresh supply of wax from within the ear. It only becomes troublesome when there is a build-up of too much wax which, if left for a long time, may harden or slip against the drum and cause hearing problems.

When you first become aware of the familiar slight 'muzziness' caused by a build-up of wax, try softening the wax with a little olive oil, at body temperature, dropped into the ears two or three times a day. Alternatively, there are special ear-wax softening drops, sometimes medicated, which your pharmacist can recommend or your doctor may prescribe – and which I prefer to olive oil. Either way, the wax may then gradually slide out on its own.

However, I must urge you to take great care with your ears – never delve inside too deeply or you could damage the drum. Do not attempt to clean or unblock your ears with cotton wool buds – you can easily abraid the skin and cause inflammation. And don't use force or instruments in the ear. Never use ear drops in an attempt to soften wax if your ears are inflamed or infected. It's not likely that there will be much wax there in any case, since wax tends to build up most in healthy ears. It's there to protect the ears, which it does admirably for most of the time in most ears and should be left alone whenever possible.

If you do use drops and after two to three days your ears still don't feel clear, consult your doctor. Your ears may need syringing with warm water.

Preparations prescribed Cerumol, Dioctyl, Waxsol

ENDOMETRIOSIS

Many women have endometriosis and don't even know they have it. Endometriosis is no more than misplaced womb lining tissue (endometrium) which has moved to another part of the body.

Each month, a woman's hormones cause a build-up in the lining of the womb, in preparation for the fertilised egg. But when there is no fertilised egg, the hormone level plummets and her period starts. Unfortunately, the same hormone which causes the womb lining to build up and then fall away, has a similar effect on the endometrium elsewhere. So, wherever the tissue has been misplaced, whether on the outside of the womb, on the ovary or Fallopian tube, a tiny bleed (like a period) occurs within the tissue.

The surrounding tissues, to which the endometriosis is attached as well as the endometriosis itself, can become inflamed. This causes swelling, pain, and within months scar tissue can be formed. The amount of pain is not always related to the extent of the disease. Symptoms can include painful periods, pain at ovulation, painful intercourse, swollen abdomen, pain before urination, loss of stale brown blood before or after periods, back pain.

Pregnancy, and regular breastfeeding, both of which prevent ovulation and therefore periods, provide a remission of symptoms.

Birth control pills or other types of hormone preparations can be prescribed to prevent periods for a time. With no period, there is no build-up of womb lining and, for the sufferer, no bleeding of the diseased tissue. When the hormone treatment is stopped after nine months, all may have quietened down so much that the symptoms may have gone. But, if symptoms persist, the gynaecologist may suggest surgery to remove some endometriosis deposits.

An example of a drug used to treat endometriosis is Primolut-N, a progestogen, whose side-effects include slight nausea, exacerbation of epilepsy and migraine. Another drug is Depo-Provera which contains medroxyprogesterone acetate. Side-effects can include transient infertility lasting up to two years or longer following continuous treatment; disruption of the normal menstrual cycle, prolonged or heavy bleeding during the first two to three cycles of treatment, back pain, weight gain and fluid retention.

Gestrinone (Dimetriose) may be prescribed. This is a synthetic steroid hormone and an antiprogestogen. It's believed to act by reducing the hormones that act upon and are produced by the ovaries. It is also thought to have a direct beneficial effect upon the endometriosis tissue itself.

Danazol (Danol) is now a popular drug. It prevents periods by hindering the production of the two hormones produced by the pituitary, which controls the ovaries. Without these hormones the endometrial sites shrivel up. It helps control pain and pelvic tenderness. Side effects can be a problem. These include weight gain, fluid retention, oily skin and an acne flare-up, nausea and muscle spasms. However, scar tissue does usually lessen and it increases the chances of a conception occuring when this is or has been hampered by the endometriosis.

Nasal sprays can also be prescribed. Suprecur (buserelin acetate), for example, is very similar to the hormones known as LHRH produced at the base of our brains – the hypothalamus. However, it competes with LHRH. When sufficient doses are used regularly, it reduces the activity of the ovaries and the concentration of the hormones they produce falls. Consequently, with this type of treatment, most women suffer menopausal symptoms – the kind they may experience when their ovaries cease to function at the time of their menopause.

Unfortunately, endometriosis isn't confined to the pelvic area. It can be found on other parts of the body. The misplaced endometrial cells were probably carried to the new site in the blood stream as a 'seed' of endometriosis. If it occurs on the skin it will look like a small spot and will bleed every month.

Many women who have endometriosis have no symptoms and it is only found when they undergo abdominal surgery. Unfortunately, for some women, hormone treatment and the occasional removal of the diseased tissue by an operation may still leave them suffering from endometriosis.

There are a number of support groups for endometriosis sufferers. With their help, women can talk with others in the same situation. It is a great comfort, not least because they are made to feel that they are not alone, especially as one of the most distressing aspects of the disease is that it can lead to infertility.

If we knew why some women develop endometriosis, we could then be able to stop it at source.

Preparations prescribed Danol, Depo-Provera, Dimetriose, Duphaston, Primolut N, Provera, Suprecur, Synarel, Utovlan, Zoladex

EPILEPSY

Epilepsy is a pattern of fits or seizures caused by an abnormal discharge of electric energy from the brain. Sufferers experience short episodes of changed behaviour or consciousness. The fits are called generalised when the whole brain is affected or if it's a partial fit it is called focal.

Most people who suffer from epilepsy are able to control their fits completely with appropriate drugs. These anti-convulsant drugs help neutralise excessive electrical activity in the brain.

Specialists are able to use precisely the right amount of medication, now that they can monitor its concentration in the body by blood tests.

There's a wide variety of drugs available for the sufferer, just as there's a wide variety of experiences of epilepsy itself, ranging from short periods of blankness all the way to full-blown convulsions, which can look very frightening indeed to someone who isn't familiar with them. The age of the sufferer and the way they respond to a drug is also taken into account when deciding upon which one.

Examples of the types of drugs used for tonic/clonic seizures (also called *grand mal*) are phenytoin (Epanutin), and phenobarbitone (Gardenal Sodium). For absence seizures (*petit mal*), which mainly affect children, ethosuximide (Emeside, Zarontin) and sodium valproate (Epilim, Orlept) are prescribed. For partial seizures, drugs used are phenytoin, phenobarbitone and carbamazepine.

The most common side-effects of these drugs are caused by the drug's action on the body's central nervous system. You won't find this surprising since these drugs are given to control the symptoms produce by this system. Dizziness, insomnia, nervousness, an occasional episode of slurred speech or mental confusion may occur, as may nausea, vomiting or rashes. Some drugs may have effects upon the blood cells, so blood tests may need to be taken from time to time to keep a check on this.

Thanks to these drugs, the outlook has never been better for those with epilepsy. It's also important for their friends and family to appreciate that epilepsy is not an illness itself, but a symptom of a condition which, in its most dramatic form, results in convulsions. In many people, there seems to be no reason for what happens; it is a little like the brain being struck by sheet lightning. But just as, often, there's no reason why these fits start, they can also disappear in some cases. For these people, the specialist will probably suggest that the medicine is decreased gradually to see how they cope. But while coming off drugs, they should continue not to drive or operate machinery.

And I would just like to put the record straight while talking about epilepsy. No objects should be jammed into a sufferer's mouth while he or she is having a fit as, during this seizure, the person cannot swallow or spit out anything – which is why saliva spills out. If a bit of tooth is chipped off by inserting an object into the mouth, this can go down into the lungs and be potentially life-threatening. Thankfully, attitudes towards those with epilepsy are changing, although perhaps not dramatically or quickly enough.

Preparations prescribed Emeside, Epanutin, Epilim, Frisium, Gardenal Sodium, Lamictal, Mysoline, Neurontin, Orlept, Prominal, Rivotril, Sabril, Tegretol, Zarontin

FLUID RETENTION

Fluid retention, or oedema, is caused by fluid leaking from the body's circulatory system. It then builds up in the body's tissue. The most usual place is the ankles, causing the ankles to become swollen and puffy. This is because the force of gravity causes it to accumulate there. If the sufferer is confined to bed, then the oedema collects in the small of the back since that is where gravity is pulling it to.

A swelling happens as a result of knocking yourself or from an injury. Fluid retention occurs as a consequence of various diseases; heart, kidney or liver disease, are examples of the more common of them.

Less serious, though sometimes most unpleasant, conditions like the irritable bowel syndrome or pre-menstrual syndrome can cause bloating – although this is not quite the same as oedema since actual fluid rarely collects around the ankles or in the back and a blood test does not confirm the changes observed with oedema.

Fluid retention can be treated by diuretics which act on the kidneys to promote urine secretion – that is, an extra output of salt and water from the body. They do this by stopping the normal retention of salt by the kidney, and this allows the excess liquid to be 'drawn' away by the salt into the urine.

Potassium levels can be lowered as a result of taking some diuretics. This can lead to weakness and confusion and the elderly are particularly at risk. Potassium supplements help to redress the balance or a potassium-sparing diuretic can be prescribed.

Preparations prescribed Diurexan, Esidrex, Frusene, Hydrosaluric, Hygroton, Kalspare, Lasix, Lasikal + K Combination Pack, Lasix Paediatric Liquid, Metenix, Midamor, Navidrex, Saluric

GOUT

Gout, or acute gouty arthritis, is a common and extremely painful form of arthritis. It's an inflammatory reaction caused by uric acid crystals deposited in the joints, which trigger a reaction in the tissue. It begins as a sensation of discomfort, rapidly developing into excruciating pain. The joint then becomes acutely inflamed and can turn bluish-red and shiny. Gout can lead to joint damage if deposits stay and build up in the joints over a number of years.

Gouty people have a faulty system for breaking down and excreting the waste products from protein food particles (purines). Normally these waste products, particularly broken-down uric acid, are passed out in our urine but in an attack of gout uric acid builds up in the blood. Most of us pass out enough of these wastes to reduce the amount in our blood and keep the levels low. People with gout have a tendency to higher levels of uric acid than normal, either because they don't pass out enough, or they produce too much. Sometimes the high levels can be caused by eating or drinking too much, so over-producing uric acid in the body.

Not everyone with higher levels of uric acid develops gout: some people may have just one or two attacks in their life while others experience repeated bouts involving joint after joint. Gout often runs in families.

If you suffer from gout drink only a moderate amount of alcohol because it can change blood uric acid levels. And it would be sensible to avoid foods high in purines such as liver, bacon, kidneys, sweetbreads, fish roe, anchovies, herrings, mackerel, mussels, sardines, yeast extracts, yeast and beers. You should also avoid overeating in general.

Drugs used to treat gout include colchicine, an old drug used since the eighteenth century and once extracted from the autumn crocus flower. Others are allopurinol, usually taken for long-term treatment to prevent recurrent attacks, (Caplenal, Hamarin, Zyloric) which stops too much acid forming in the first place; and probenecid (Benemid) which helps the kidneys to increase the amount excreted and so aids the prevention of further attacks.

Non-steroidal anti-inflammatory drugs used in the treatment of arthritis may be prescribed to relieve the pain and inflammation. Indomethacin, azapropazone and naproxen are most frequently used (see ARTHRITIS, page 22).

Preparations prescribed Anturan, Arthroxen, Benemid, Caplenal, Clinoril, Clinoril 200, Diclomax Retard, Hamarin, Indocid, Naprosyn, Pranoxen Continus, Rheumox 600, Zyloric

HERPES (Genital)

Herpes is caused by a herpes simplex virus transferred from one infected person to another during sex. And there is no magic cure. Just like a cold sore on the lips, caused by a very similar virus, it cannot be cured as such.

This makes it sound frightening. Fortunately, however, complications, such as infections of the urethra and deeper tissues, are very rare and only occur as part of an initial attack. Inconvenient and distressing though herpes may be, it is rarely a life-threatening disease.

If you suffer from herpes, take reassurance in the fact that attacks become less and less frequent with every year that passes. Many people suffer only one attack while others have to put up with it for years. But most report that it stops as suddenly as it starts.

It's essential for any man or woman who has herpes to insist on wearing a condom during sex, especially if they suspect an attack is coming on – or better still to avoid sex altogether. While there is no cast-iron guarantee, the passing on of herpes between attacks is unlikely. But I would advise herpes sufferers to use condoms even when symptoms aren't present.

After an attack, the virus lies dormant (or 'nests') in the nerves of the genital area. Then, when the body's immune system – that's its disease defence system – is below par, the infection can erupt again. So it's important to obtain treatment as soon as herpes is suspected, to minimise the symptoms. The most effective drug available to do this is acyclovir (Zovirax) in cream or tablet form which helps the body's own defences to fight the virus (see also COLD SORES, page 40). Skin rashes have been reported in a few patients receiving Zovirax oral formulations, as well as some reports of gastrointestinal disturbances.

Another anti-viral drug used to treat herpes is inosine pranobex (Imunovir). Side-effects with this are rare and usually shortlived. The only commonly associated adverse effects are elevated serum and urinary concentrations of uric acid. These return to normal once treatment is withdrawn.

Preparations prescribed Imunovir, Zovirax

HAY FEVER

Hay fever is an allergic reaction which occurs in people who are particularly sensitive to pollen or spores released into the air by trees, grasses or moulds. Its medical name is seasonal allergic rhinitis and it is one of the most common allergies known. It is estimated that between six and 12 million people in the UK suffer – most between the ages of 10 and 40, with about one in six teenagers affected. It is also estimated that four million working days are lost during June and July alone through hay fever.

Hay fever strictly refers to an allergy to grass pollen, but the term is often used to cover allergy to pollen from plants, shrubs and trees. Pollens released in spring are usually from trees, whilst in the summer flowers, grass or weed pollens are released. In the autumn the symptoms are usually caused by pollen from autumn-flowering plants and the spores of some fungi. The sufferer's body reacts to pollen as though it were a dangerous threat like a germ, and does all it can to get rid of it by releasing a chemical called histamine. Histamine causes inflammation and irritation of the mucous membranes of the eyes, nose and ear passages. The eyes then water in an effort to wash away the pollen and the running nose and sneezing help eject pollen from the nose. Hay fever can also cause drowsiness.

Hay fever sufferers are most at risk between May and September, when the 'pollen count' (the level of pollen in the air) is at its highest. So listen to the pollen count forecasts broadcast daily on television and local radio or check the weather reports in a newspaper. A pollen count of 50 grains per cubic metre is enough to set most sufferers sneezing. The pollen count will be high on warm, dry and windy days because pollen released from grasses and trees is carried upwards by warm air. Also, warm, dry conditions are needed for pollen to be released in the first place.

Symptoms are often more severe in the morning, when pollen is released and carried upwards as the air temperature rises. They then become worse again in the evening as the temperature drops and the pollen grains drift back down.

There is no cure for hay fever, although nasal sprays available on prescription are very helpful. Your GP may prescribe an antihistamine nasal spray such as Rhinolast (azelastine hydrochloride) for example, which both blocks the action of the pollen as well as enhancing the effects that the local tissues have in overcoming them. It's a new kind of antihistamine which patients find helpful in easing congestion, sneezing and nasal itching, discharge and swelling.

Steroid drops could be prescribed. They are thought to be one of the most effective measures when managing an allergy such as hay fever. They damp down the allergic response and cut down on any inflammation and swelling. Beconase Nasal Spray (beclomethasone dipropionate), for example, is a popular choice. Rhinocort (budesonide) is another example. To get the most out of this kind of treatment you need to use the spray regularly.

Mast cell stabilisers which help control nasal symptoms by preventing allergic reactions are another option. Rynacrom Nasal Spray (sodium cromoglycate) can be used to prevent symptoms developing of both hay fever and perennial rhinitis. Since therapy is essentially preventive, it's important that you maintain regular dosage, rather than using the drops to deal with symptoms once they develop. Side-effects of sprays can be irritation of the nasal mucosa and a taste disturbance.

Antihistamines can be prescribed for hay fever and there are many different types available. An antihistamine such as promethazine (Phenergan) is a powerful long-acting antihistamine with additional anti-emetic, anticholinergic and sedative/calming effects. Most common side-effects can include drowsiness, dizziness, restlessness, headaches, nightmares, tiredness and disorientation. Piriton (chlorpheniramine maleate) can also cause drowsiness, impaired reactions and dizziness.

Newer antihistamines astemizole (Hismanal), terfenadine (Triludan), loratidine (Clarityn), acrivastine (Semprex) and cetirizine (Zirtek) can be tried. They don't have the sedative side-effects of promethazine. But care should be taken initially, as with all drugs taken for the first time, because there may be rare cases when the patient reacts badly. For most relief, antihistamines should be started as soon as the first symptoms occur.

The main side-effect of the older antihistamines is sedation. Otherwise they were relatively side-effect free. The newer ones do not sedate much, if at all, and other side-effects, such as nausea or headache are rare.

There are many self-help measures you can take to relieve the symptoms of hay fever. Wearing plain glasses or sunglasses can prevent much of the eye irritation, by stopping pollen grains entering the eyes. Keep windows and doors closed, especially when lawns are being mowed. Stay away from pets if they have been outside. Try to plan your day to avoid being outdoors in the morning and evening when pollen counts are at their highest. Don't go on country walks and avoid parks or gardens on warm and sunny days, or, if this is impossible, wash your hair afterwards. Keep car windows and air vents closed when you're out driving. Don't smoke, because this causes further irritation to those susceptible to allergies.

Preparations prescribed Beconase, Clarityn, Daneral, Dexa-Rhinaspray, Dimotane, Flixonase, Galpseud, Hismanal, Opticrom, Periactin, Phenergan, Piriton, Primalan, Pro-Actidil, Rhinocort, Rhinolast, Rynacrom, Semprex, Sudafed, Tavegil, Thephorin, Tinset, Triludan, Vibrocil, Zirtek

HEADACHE

Headaches are an extremely common complaint, afflicting one person in three at least once a year, though some people do tend to suffer more than others. In fact, although we tend to use the word headache to describe any pain in the head, there are probably more than 100 different types of headache and they vary in intensity and location. Some develop gradually and clear up after an hour or two or a walk in the fresh air. Others can be extremely severe and can last more than 24 hours.

Two of the commonest types of headache are migraine, a severe, recurring headache (see page 106) and tension headache, sometimes known as muscle contraction headache.

With migraine, the pain is usually one sided and can be accompanied by other symptoms such as loss of appetite, nausea or vomiting. In a tension headache, the whole head throbs and feels as though there's a weight on top of it or a tight band around it. The pain is usually dull and persistent, originating in the muscles of the scalp. The tension headache is the most common symptom presented to a general practitioner and no one knows the cause, or why some people get a headache when they are emotionally upset and some don't.

Different sorts of headache can also be brought on by other factors – drinking too much alcohol, sinusitis, anxiety or being in an overheated room or smoky atmosphere are all common triggers. They may be the result of muscle strain in your neck, especially if the headache comes on after you have been reading or doing close work like sewing. You can become tense from concentrating for too long or from sitting in an awkward position.

For most minor headaches, it is worth trying the following self-help measures. Take the recommended dose of a mild painkiller such as aspirin or paracetamol. For best results, take the painkiller as soon as you feel the headache coming on. Drink plenty of water or other non-alcoholic, clear drinks. Rest in a quiet, darkened room may also be soothing and a warm bath will sometimes relieve tension.

Fortunately, most headaches are not a sign of serious disease, but if your headache is particularly severe; if it's accompanied by misty or blurred vision, nausea or vomiting; if there's no satisfactory explanation for a headache that is continuous or getting worse after three days, or comes back several times in the course of a week; or if you have injured your head during the past few days, you should consult your doctor for advice. See PAINKILLERS page 121.

HEAD LICE AND PUBIC LICE

Once you get head lice, they won't let go until you do something about it! They're tiny brown insects with six short, stubbly legs. They're about the size of a pin head and live on human heads, laying six to eight eggs a day of a creamy-brown colour. They turn white when the baby louse, called a nymph, has hatched. The remaining pearly white husk is commonly known as a nit. At this stage it is a harmless shell.

The eggs are attached near the base of the hair shaft – a favourite spot is around the ears. Each louse takes two weeks to mature and lives for 20 to 30 days if undetected. The lice feed on blood, using their specially developed mouth-parts to pierce the scalp. They even inject a local anaesthetic into the scalp to prevent their host feeling any pain, and an anticoagulant to stop the blood clotting, thus making it easier for them to feed! They can eventually make your head feel very itchy because, after about 10,000 bites, your immune system becomes understandably irritated. And you don't feel well either, which is how the phrase 'I feel lousy' originated.

To check whether someone has head lice, dampen their hair and then bend their head over a plain sheet of paper. Comb the hair thoroughly to see whether any insects drop out. Quickly part the hair to look out for moving lice. A magnifying glass will help.

Head lice can sometimes be a problem among schoolchildren. That's because the head louse has never had it so good. We and our children are healthier and cleaner that we have ever been, and the head louse loves it. Clean, healthy heads provide it with the perfect environment for perpetuating its lifestyle. Every time a clean-headed child comes into contact with another child's head as they play, the head louse moves from one head to another. Head lice can't jump or fly, nor do they survive in bedding, furniture or clothes. The only way they can be passed on is by close head contact – a single louse can visit several heads in one day just be walking from one to another.

So if you or your children have head lice, please don't worry or feel ashamed about going to see your doctor.

More than a million people a year in the UK get head lice, so there's no point in being embarrassed about it. It's also pretty well impossible to prevent children catching head lice from each other, as it's nothing to do with them being dirty or neglected. Like chickenpox, it's just another of those things children are likely to catch once they start mixing with others.

Pubic lice (commonly called crabs) are passed on during sexual intercourse. Irritation and itching in the pubic region can be extremely uncomfortable and intense. The lice can often be seen at a glance and look like tiny scabs.

Your GP can prescribe one of a variety of lotions and shampoos for head lice. You can also buy them without a prescription at your pharmacist. Some of them, such as one containing carbaryl (Carylderm) or malathion (Derbac-M), will also be suitable for getting rid of pubic lice. When applying a shampoo or lotion, remember to ensure that no part of the scalp or pubic hair is left uncovered; pay particular attention to the nape of the neck and behind the ears when dealing with head lice.

There are three main insecticides in use that kill head lice and their eggs – carbaryl, pyrethroids (phenothrin, permethrin) and malathion. They are all equally effective if used according to the directions. But health authorities usually change their recommendations for louse treatment preparations every two to three years to prevent the lice building up a resistance to them.

Bear in mind, too, that should a member of your family need treatment, you must treat the whole family – parents, grandparents, even lodgers – and then check them once a week to ensure they're still clear. This applies equally to pubic lice since these can be passed on by children who may share a bed or if they regularly get into other beds of family members. The lice can remain for a very short time on the bedding. However, the main way in which pubic lice are passed on is by a regular bed partner, especially one who is in intimate contact.

Make sure your children's friends don't have lice either or there could be a risk of re-infection. It's wise – if not essential – to inform your child's school if you discover head lice.

Then, after treatment, encourage all your family to comb their hair thoroughly every day, since the female louse – and there are many more of them than the male – must cling on to two hairs to survive; as combing or brushing separates the hair, the louse will then die. Once dead, it falls off harmlessly.

Preparations prescribed Carylderm, Clinicide, Derbac-C, Derbac-M, Full Marks, Lyclear, Prioderm, Suleo-C, Suleo-M

HIATUS HERNIA

See INDIGESTION AND RELATED PROBLEMS page 96

HIGH BLOOD PRESSURE

Judging by the great number and variety of different preparations to treat high blood pressure it's obviously a pretty common problem. Something like one in five people are now on medication for high blood pressure. Yet hypertension, to call it by its medical name, is not a disease in itself. But having it can make you more vulnerable to strokes, heart and kidney disease. When your heart beats it causes a surge of blood which raises the blood pressure.

I'm often asked what an abnormal blood pressure reading is. Well, the first part of the reading denotes the pressure in the main arteries and heart as they pulse or beat (systolic). The second reading is the pressure between the beats (diastolic).

A low blood pressure found during a routine check is usually a health benefit as it indicates the heart and blood vessels are not under stress, and so the person should live longer than average as a result. Between the ages of 15 and 40, measurements ranging from 90/60 to 50/90 can be considered normal when the person is at rest. A rough rule easy to remember is that normal systolic pressure should generally be 100 plus your age, and the diastolic pressure less than 90.

Blood pressure can increase quite naturally as we get older. In a middle-aged person, for example, a reading of 160/100 could be considered normal enough not to require any treatment if that person is otherwise fit and healthy.

In this instance, the doctor would feel that the risks of constantly raised blood pressure – i.e. an increased possibility of strokes, as well as heart and kidney problems – would be no greater than the risk of side-effects from treatment that might upset the body's delicate chemical balance.

From time to time, blood pressure levels will be raised considerably above normal, during bouts of physical exertion or emotional anxiety. This is the body's way of preparing itself for action, or of dealing with a threat.

But the good news is that high blood pressure can at least be controlled. For the most part, people who have high blood pressure do not have any symptoms. Often, they only know they're hypertensive – have high blood pressure – when a doctor tests their blood pressure, perhaps because a life assurance policy requires it.

Most doctors also fully appreciate the need to treat blood pressure by natural means whenever possible. These include advising the patient to lose weight, give up smoking, cut down on salt and on fatty foods and avoid excessive alcohol, and to try to take some form of exercise.

In this country, we all, on average, eat far too much salt. This is because our tastebuds are used to it. Now, while it's difficult to prove it is actually causing harm – though I believe it is – there is proof that for someone whose blood pressure is already too high, excess salt will make it even higher. Consequently, the chance of a stroke – a burst blood vessel in the brain which can cause paralysis – becomes greater.

Just by eating a balanced diet, you will take in more than enough salt for health. Pre-cooked and processed foods nearly always have extra salt added. So avoiding those is a help, as is not adding salt to cooking or at the table. This will cut the average salt intake by a quarter.

Relaxation techniques can also be a great help. Stress does make blood pressure zoom up. A doctor will take tests to check whether a patient's high blood pressure is permanently high and needs medicine. Before medical treatment he or she will also establish that the individual's blood pressure remains at a high level under normal circumstances. And he or she will determine whether the organs of the body have suffered as a result of the increased blood pressure.

Abnormally high blood pressure can affect the heart, making it larger as it endeavours to cope with the strain of pumping the blood around the body under higher pressure. It can affect the kidneys in extreme cases, causing them to fail.

But for the majority of sufferers, there is one simple message. Once it's determined their blood pressure is high and no primary or treatable cause can be found, they should expect to remain on their doctor's medicines forever.

The four main groups of medicines used to treat high blood pressure, and which all act in different ways, are diuretics (water pills), betablockers (these act on the nerves which control circulation), ACE inhibitors (which block an enzyme which increases blood pressure) and a calcium antagonist (a medicine which alters the way minerals enter and leave the body cells). Doctors have found that most often an individual's blood pressure can be controlled by using a combination of two of these medicines in smaller doses than would be needed if one was used by itself. What's more, having four efficient types of medicines at their disposal means doctors can choose the ones that best suit each individual's body and way of life.

The side-effects of diuretics and tablets to treat high blood pressure can include low potassium levels (particularly in the elderly), mild dizziness and mild stomach upsets. If you are taking medication for high blood pressure you should always let your doctor know if you experience fast heart beats, or palpitations, swelling of the ankles, feet or lower legs, skin troubles such as a rash or itching for the first time, muscle pain or cramps, any unusual bleeding or bruising, or any yellow discoloration of the whites of your eyes and skin.

Preparations prescribed Accupro, Accuretic, Adizem, Aldactide, Apresoline, Arelix, Beta-Adalat, Betaloc, Blocadren, Calcilat, Carace, Cardinol, Catapres, Celectol, Co-Betaloc, Decaserpyl, Declinax, Diurexan, Emcor, Esidrex, Geangin, Hydromet, Hydrosaluric, Hygroton, Hytrin, Inderal, Inderetic, Inderex, Innovace, Ismelin, Kalspare, Kalten, Kerlone, Lasipressin, Lopresor, Lopresoretic, Metenix, Mudocren, Navispare, Nifensar, Saluric, Secadrex, Sectral, Slow-Trasicor, Tenif, Teneroet, Tenoret, Tenormin, Tildiem, Totamol, Trasicor, Trasidrex, Tritace, Univer, Vascace, Viskaldix, Visken, Zestoretic, Zestril

HIGH CHOLESTEROL

First, I'll explain a little more about cholesterol. It is one of three fats in the blood and comes in two forms – the 'good' type, HDL, and the 'bad' type, LDL. Triglycerides are the third fat circulating in the body.

A raised cholesterol level in the blood is one of the most widely recognised causes of coronary artery and other heart conditions. What's more, it's not only the heart that can be affected.

What happens is that the cholesterol is deposited just under the lining of the heart, its arteries, and all the arteries in the body. This restricts the flow of blood and so can cause coronary thrombosis – a heart attack. It can also weaken the arteries to the extent that they burst. If this happens in the brain, it's called a stroke; if it happens in the big arteries of the heart, it's a dissecting aneurysm.

That's the bad news. On the good side, reducing the level of cholesterol to a normal blood level – especially if it's done in a way that increases the proportion of good cholesterol (HDL) – can reverse much, or all, of the damage that's been done.

If you are currently suffering from a higher than normal level of cholesterol there are three simple steps to put it right.

1. Slim down to your ideal weight.
2. Reduce the amount of all fats in your diet, especially the saturated variety, usually of animal origin.
3. Take more regular exercise.

It's also a good idea to eat proportionately more unsaturated fats and oils, such as cod liver, olive and corn oils.

If a blood test indicates that your cholesterol level is higher than average, don't be alarmed, but do consult your doctor.

Some people inherit the condition and when this is the cause of the problem, it's not always possible to reduce the high levels by natural means, so drugs may be required. These lower the cholesterol levels and may have the effect of reducing any deposits that may have already formed.

Groups of drugs used include bile acid sequestrants – cholestyramine (such as Questran A) and colestipol (such as Colestid). These lower the blood cholesterol levels by preventing the bile acids (rich in cholesterol) from being absorbed from the bowel (into which they are secreted by the liver) and taken into the bloodstream, as they are under normal circumstances.

Fibric acid drugs (also called isobutyric acid derivatives) reduce high blood fat levels. Examples are clofibrate (Atromid-S), bezafibrate (Bezalip Mono), fenofibrate (Lipantil) and gemfibrozil (Lopid).

Then there's the nicotinic acid type – nicotinic acid (niacin, which can cause flushing and headache), acipimox (Olbetam) and nicofuranose (Bradilan). Acipimox inhibits the breakdown of the body's fatty acid stores and has a beneficial reducing effect upon the worst kind of cholesterol – the very low density kind, as it's known.

There's also a newer group of drugs which tend to be used for those people who don't have much success with other medicines, pravastatin (Lipostat) and simvastatin (Zocor). These tend to inhibit the enzymes – the chemical enhancers – which are essential for the formation of blood cholesterol. When effective the production of cholesterol, and hence the concentration in the blood, falls.

Drugs used to treat high cholesterol can cause a variety of side-effects including gastro-intestinal upsets, flushes, rashes, constipation and headaches.

Preparations prescribed Atromid, Bradilan, Colestid, Lipantil, Lipostat, Lopid, Olbetam, Questran-A, Zocor

HORMONE REPLACEMENT THERAPY

In my opinion, hormone replacement therapy (HRT), supplementing the hormone oestrogen which women stop producing during the menopause, is one of the greatest medical breakthroughs of the past 20 years or so, and the treatment is expected to become a lot more common in the next decade. I, for one, believe HRT will greatly benefit women who are in their middle and later years.

While only one in five women experiences excessive menopausal symptoms like hot flushes and depression, at least another one or two in five will suffer less severe characteristics – emotional and social, as well as physical – which they don't necessarily relate to the menopause until they've tried HRT and discovered the difference in the way they feel. Of course, HRT will not necessarily overcome the apprehension felt at the passing of the years, but it does help a great number of women to feel more optimistic about the prospect, and to have more confidence in themselves.

It's not just the symptoms of the menopause that will be relieved, either. An unacceptable proportion of women in later years develop osteoporosis – commonly known as brittle bones – and HRT can prevent this. Osteoporosis causes not only thinning of the bones, but also more distressing changes, like the spine bending to produce a hump at the top. This causes the woman to lose height, and she may end up being several inches shorter than before.

HRT can be taken in several ways: by pill; by a sticky plaster-type patch stuck to a fleshy area and replaced every three days; or by 'injected' pellets (implants), which last up to three months before they need replacing. Another option is by creams placed in the vagina. The latter, however, are more often used for the treatment of a dry and itchy vagina – that is, a symptom of the menopause – rather than to replace the body's overall supply of oestrogen.

Patches should be applied to a clean, dry, hairless area of skin below the waistline, preferably on the buttocks where body movements don't make your skin wrinkle and there's less chance of friction from clothing working the patch loose. A new area of skin should be selected for each fresh application. Patches should not be applied on or near the breasts. Applied in this way, the hormones will then pass continuously through your skin and into your body. There can sometimes be some mild irritation from patches, perhaps some itching and reddening of the skin. This usually disappears in three to four days.

Women who've had hysterectomies will be given only oestrogen. Otherwise, doctors recommend that patients take two female hormones during the month. The second one, progestogen, induces a light period. The amounts of oestrogen and progestogen are balanced carefully so that they are right for the individual. However, recently, a new HRT pill has been introduced, which a woman can take every day, without a period following. It's called Livial.

I think the day will come when HRT will be compared favourably with other replacement medicines that are required when the body fails to produce its own – such as the thyroid hormone and even insulin, with its life-enhancing properties for the diabetic.

One disadvantage of HRT is that most women will have menstrual periods and even monthly breast tenderness. Some women may feel a little sick or get headaches during the first few weeks of treatment. Leg cramps are also quite common. These effects happen as your body adjusts to having a regular supply of hormones again, and usually disappear after the first few weeks of treatment. If they continue for more than three months discuss the problem with your doctor. But the advantages are stronger bones and muscles, better looking skin, the continuity of normal vaginal secretions, no hot flushes and a reduced risk of heart disease.

Studies show that both heart disease and female cancers of the uterus and ovaries are less frequent in women taking HRT. Because many, if not most, cancers of the breast can be treated by stopping a woman's body from producing oestrogen, or blocking its action, it has been suggested that HRT, which relies on oestrogen, could be a 'cause' of breast cancer. The expert researchers continue to debate the subject but the evidence has not been seen to be sufficient to alter the recommendation for HRT in a fit woman – the advantages appear to heavily outweigh any potential disadvantages.

It's likely that, in the future, once started, many women will continue to take HRT for the rest of their natural life. At present, it is expected that they will continue to take it for about ten years after they reach the menopause.

Unfortunately, HRT isn't suitable for everyone and it's extremely important your doctor is aware of your full medical history before prescribing. It's not suitable for a woman who has had recent breast cancer, severe jaundice, some forms of thrombosis, womb-lining cancer or when a woman might be, or is, pregnant or breastfeeding. Endometriosis, fibroids, gall bladder disease, undiagnosed vaginal bleeding and otosclerosis (an ear disorder) are other conditions where HRT may be inadvisable.

Preparations prescribed Combined preparations: Climagest, Cyclo-Progynova, Estracombi, Estrapak, Livial, Nuvelle, Prempak C, Trisequens. Oestrogen preparations: Climaval, Estraderm, Harmogen, Hormonin, Oestradiol Implants, Ortho-Dienoestrol, Ortho-Gynest, Premarin, Progynova, Zumenon.

HEARTBURN

See INDIGESTION AND RELATED PROBLEMS (below)

HIVES

See URTICARIA page 160

INDIGESTION AND RELATED PROBLEMS

Symptoms of indigestion, usually felt just below or behind the breast bone, vary from an uncomfortable feeling of fullness to nausea, pain, belching, heartburn and wind. Most people will suffer from indigestion from time to time. Often there is no recognisable pattern to the symptoms, but they may be noticeably worse just before or after a meal. Nearly one person in ten takes a remedy for some form of indigestion every day and of these, one in three will have had symptoms for ten years or more. Three out of four sufferers never consult a doctor. The problem becomes more common after middle age, particularly in those who are overweight. Sensitive, anxious people are also more prone to indigestion, as anxiety increases the output of acid secretions in the stomach.

The most common form of indigestion is called heartburn, an apt name as it well describes the symptoms – waves of burning pain behind the breast bone and sometimes a burning feeling in the throat. The pain can be mistaken for heart pain (angina), but in fact angina improves with rest, whereas heartburn is usually worse when the sufferer is lying down. It is easy to see why when we look more closely at what causes it.

The stomach produces strong acid secretions which help to digest and sterilise our food. The stomach lining has a mucous coating which protects it against the acid, but the oesophagus – the gullet down which food passes from the mouth to the stomach – does not. Normally a ring of muscle – the cardiac sphincter – at the bottom end of the oesophagus acts like a trapdoor and prevents acid rising up from the stomach. Sometimes, however, if the muscle becomes a little lax, for instance as it often does during pregnancy, small amounts of acid will enter the lower part of the oesophagus – a process known as reflux. It is normal for this to happen occasionally and the saliva we are constantly swallowing will usually be enough to neutralise the acid without symptoms being caused. Also, contractions of the muscle walls of the gullet prevent the acid rising by keeping food and saliva moving downwards.

However, if reflux occurs too often, the oesophagus will gradually become inflamed and painful as the acid burns into the tissues. This inflammation is called oesophagitis. Without effective treatment the lining of the gullet can eventually become ulcerated and constricted by scarring so that swallowing food can be difficult. Other changes in the cells may also develop in time. It is important, therefore, to treat heartburn early on to prevent oesophagitis progressing.

Similar symptoms can be produced by an hiatus

hernia. A hernia occurs when tissue or an organ bulges out of its usual position. The most common sort arises in the groin when some of the abdominal contents squeeze through a hole and protrude into the groin. It's true that this sort of hernia is more usually found in men, partly because it's often linked to lifting and other strenuous activity. An hiatus hernia, however, is a lot more common in women. The symptoms arise because part of the stomach is able to 'herniate' upwards into the chest, with the result that the irritant gastric juices can seep through to the gullet. The lining of the gullet, or oesophagus, is not protected against the acids and enzymes of the digestive juices, with the result that it becomes inflamed. Once this condition is diagnosed there are several medicines that can be prescribed to help treat hiatus hernia (also known as reflux oesophagitis).

A medicine such as Gaviscon eases the pain resulting from the reflux of gastric acid and bile into the oesophagus by suppressing the reflux itself. It reacts with gastric acid to produce a floating viscous gel of near neutral pH which effectively impedes reflux. In severe cases the gel itself may be refluxed into the oesophagus, where it protects the inflamed mucosa, so allowing healing to take place and preventing any more inflammation.

Another useful medicine is Algicon. It can be useful in heartburn associated with gastric reflux, reflux oesophagitis, hiatus hernia, pregnancy and hyperacidity which also works in a similar way. Other medicines used to treat indigestion are called antacids (a large selection can be bought from your pharmacist). There are several types which can be prescribed, for example, aluminium hydroxide, calcium carbonate, magnesium hydroxide, magnesium trisilicate, hydrotalcite, and sodium bicarbonate. Some antacids are more effective than others and often it's a question of working out which one suits you best. For instance, magnesium hydroxide can take a while to have any effect but relief is fairly long lasting.

Some remedies – those containing calcium, for instance – wear off quickly, and by over-neutralising the existing acid in the stomach, may have the rebound effect of actually stimulating further acid production. Also, the calcium and sodium salts contained in some antacids will be absorbed into the bloodstream, and this is undesirable in the longer term.

Remember that all antacids can interfere with the absorption of other drugs, so remind your doctor if you are taking any other medicines.

Indigestion can have other causes: secretions such as pepsin (an enzyme which aids digestion) and bile from the liver (which helps digest fatty foods) are also capable of irritating the vulnerable stomach. Anxious people will often, unconsciously, swallow more air with their food and eat faster than others, causing distension, a rumbling stomach and belching. This type of indigestion may be relieved by learning techniques for relaxation (with the help of cassettes, for example) and by eating smaller, more frequent meals, slowly.

Many people think that eating greasy, rich or spicy foods, or eating too much too quickly, are the main causes of heartburn. In fact, although these do play a part, smoking more than ten cigarettes a day and drinking heavily are the most common causes, as both of these relax the cardiac sphincter and therefore make reflux more likely. Bouts of indigestion are therefore sometimes a warning signal that the body is being abused. Alcohol, especially on an empty stomach, and smoking both stimulate acid production and inflame the stomach.

Some drugs – antibiotics, iron tablets and aspirin, for example – can also inflame the oesophagus and cause heartburn, especially if they are taken with too little fluid or just before going to bed. Citrus fruits, chocolate, coffee and, perhaps surprisingly, peppermint are other possible culprits.

A sensitivity to certain foods, such as sugar and milk, can also cause unpleasant indigestion, as can fatty foods for some people. Cutting down on stimulants and avoiding foods found to aggravate the symptoms will, in this case, usually relieve them.

Indigestion and heartburn are also common during pregnancy. Being overweight, large meals and lack of exercise are other predisposing factors. If indigestion or heartburn is worrying or persistent, a doctor's examination and perhaps some special investigations may be necessary to exclude underlying causes such as hiatus hernia, peptic ulcer or gall bladder trouble.

In most cases of occasional indigestion, self-help measures can help. One easy, do-it-yourself aid for heartburn is to prop up the head of your bed by about six inches; perhaps you can use several pillows to raise yourself, too. That way the burning juices are less likely to flow upwards. If you're overweight, a calorie-controlled diet can help, as any excess tissue can press on the stomach and push the acid upwards. For the same reason, when you need to pick up something from the floor, bend from the knees rather than the waist. Eat slowly, sitting upright, not slouched in front of the television, and chew your food thoroughly before swallowing. Don't wear tight belts or corsets, as they increase pressure on the stomach.

Preparations prescribed Algicon, Alu-cap, Aluhyde, aluminium hydroxide, calcium carbonate, Dyspamet, Galenamet, Gastrobid, Gastron, Gaviscon, Infant Gaviscon, Kolanticon, Maalox, magnesium hydroxide, magnesium trisilicate, Mucogel, Pyrogastrone, Tagamet, Topal

INSOMNIA

See SLEEPLESSNESS page 145

INTERTRIGO

Intertrigo is an inflammation of large, moist skin surfaces that are in close contact. The area becomes red, angry and moist. It is most common in babies (in the skin creases of the groin), the elderly (in women under pendulous breasts) and the obese – where an 'apron' of abdomen may become so large that it hangs down and an area of intertrigo forms underneath. Your doctor may prescribe an ointment to reduce inflammation (a mild topical steroid such as hydrocortisone, Hydrocortisyl or Quinocort) and to help heal the infected area, or one combined with an antibacterial agent such as Synalar N or with the addition of an antifungal agent such as Synalar C. But to make sure the problem doesn't reccur it is important to maintain good standards of hygiene.

Preparations prescribed Hydrocortisyl Skin Cream and Ointment, Quinocort Cream, Synalar C or N Cream or ointment, Tinaderm-M Cream.

IRON DEFICIENCY IN PREGNANCY

It's thought that during pregnancy one third of a woman's iron reserves pass over to her baby. This is because iron is an essential component of muscle, blood and tissue cells and the developing foetus is building these up at an astonishing rate. To counteract this it's important to eat a well-balanced diet with plenty of iron rich foods (see ANAEMIA, page 12). Women whose iron levels are low can be prescribed various supplements to prevent iron-deficiency anaemia. An example is Pregaday which contains iron and folic acid. These tablets are usually given at about the thirteenth week of pregnancy either as a routine measure, in some instances, or because the haemoglobin level of the blood is less than 75% of normal. A low haemoglobin level makes the blood less efficient in carrying oxygen, so that at very low levels (50% or less) the sufferer will quickly become breathless on exertion and will feel very tired and lethargic. At even lower levels, the heart, too, may become far less efficient, so increasing the breathlessness and other symptoms.

Iron is an essential component of haemoglobin, and folic acid (a component of the B vitamin group) is essential for the production of blood. As with most other medicines, iron supplements are undesirable during the first three months of pregnancy.

Sometimes women experience nausea and gastro-intestinal irritation when they take some – not all – iron supplements.

Preparations prescribed Ferrograd Folic, Ferrocontin Folic Continus Tablets, Folicin, Meterfolic, Pregaday, Slow-Fe Folic

IRRITABLE BOWEL SYNDROME

Irritable bowel syndrome is a very common disorder which causes pain to be felt anywhere in the abdomen, which can move from one side to another. It can also cause a bloated feeling. Despite experiencing often severe pain, people suffering from irritable bowel syndrome can look very well. The pain is caused by spasm in the muscles of the bowel walls, causing a kind of cramp.

It helps to eat more fibre and bulking agents can be prescribed as well. Fybogel, for instance, contains isphaghula husk which helps restore regular bowel function and is capable of absorbing up to 40 times its own weight in water.

Treatment can also include the prescribing of anti-spasmodics which either relax muscle or are anti-cholinergic, that is, inhibit the action of acetylcholine. That means the transmission of nerve signals to the bowel wall are cut down and so reduce spasm.

An antispasmodic such as mebeverine hydrochloride (Colofac) is helpful. It has a direct action on the smooth muscle of the gastrointestinal tract, relieving spasm without affecting normal gut motility. It can help alleviate symptoms such as colicky abdominal pain and cramps, persistent non-specific diarrhoea (with or without alternating diarrhoea), constipation and flatulence. A new product, Fybogel Mebeverine, contains ispaghula husk and mebeverine hydrochloride, a combination treatment. Another example of a combination treatment is Alvercol which contains sterculia (a water absorbing vegetable gum) and alverine citrate (an antispasmodic agent). Peppermint oil capsules (Mintec, for example) can help relax gastrointestinal smooth muscle and relieve flatulence and colic.

Irritable bowels are undoubtedly made worse if the sufferer is tense and anxious. Indeed, almost everyone who is suddenly anxious can experience an unpleasant feeling of butterflies in their abdomen. An irritable bowel is that sort of feeling but with pain being the most noticeable element – sometimes a dull, persistent, ache, sometimes a dull colicky pain. In nine out of ten sufferers it's combined with constipation. One in ten will have diarrhoea – or at least pass several motions per day.

Preparations prescribed Alvercol, Colofac, Colpermin, Colven, Fybogel, Fybogel Mebeverine, Mintec, Pro-Banthine, Spasmonal, Trifyba

KIDNEY INFECTIONS

Most of us with healthy, functioning kidneys take them very much for granted, not fully realising the complex and vital task they perform.

Each kidney is composed of a million tiny filter units, or nephrons as they are called. Every five minutes of the day and night all the blood circulating in our body (about eight pints altogether) passes through the kidneys to be cleansed. Any chemical impurities resulting from food digestion are filtered out and excreted in the urine. Nutrients, necessary body salts and water are reabsorbed.

Repeated urinary infections, if not properly treated can cause permanent kidney damage. So your doctor's advice should be sought if you have symptoms of such an infection. These will include pain or a burning sensation on passing urine, a dull ache or sharp pain either side of the spine in the back, just below the ribs, or just an ill feeling, maybe with a temperature. Treatment is usually by antibiotic, see page 17.

MALARIA

Malaria is a disease found in certain tropical countries and causes bouts of fever (with shivering attacks), headache and muscle pains. At times it can be serious but if you are travelling to a relevant country, don't panic. In the main it can be prevented by taking anti-malarial tablets and commonsense measures.

Malaria occurs when small parasites are passed from one person to another by the bites of certain (infected) female mosquitoes. If you are planning a holiday, or business trip, to a malaria-prone area, do seek the advice of your doctor or pharmacist as the choice of tablets does depend on the country and how long you are planning to visit. And if you are prescribed anti-malarial tablets (as with any other medicine) make sure you follow directions to the letter.

You'll need to take the full course – and remember that as no anti-malaria medicine is 100 per cent effective, there is a small risk that malaria can develop during or after preventive medication. You may be prescribed drugs such as chloroquine (Avloclor, Nivaquine, for example), proguanil (Paludrine), sulfadoxine combined with pyrimethamine (Fansidar) among others.

Side-effects of anti-malaria drugs include rashes, gastrointestinal upsets and sometimes blood disorders.

When you do travel abroad, make sure you sleep in a room that is screened against mosquitoes or that you use a mosquito net (preferably one that has been treated with an insect repellant) over the bed. Check for holes in the net, and be sure to tuck the edges under the mattress before nightfall. Use insect repellants, ointments, lotions and sprays to deter mosquitoes. In the evening, cover arms and legs with light coloured, long-sleeved clothes and trousers, and use an insect repellent. Anklets are also available which have been treated with repellent. Vapourising electric 'mats', mosquito coils or tablets can be used around exposed areas of the body (ankles and feet). Electronic buzzers are considered ineffective.

Preparations prescribed Avloclor, Daraprim, Fansidar, Lariam, Maloprim, Nivaquine, Paludrine

MENOPAUSE, THE

The menopause, referred to as the change, or the change of life, comes about when the ovaries stop producing the female hormone oestrogen.

The most common symptoms are hot flushes and night sweats. These can be accompanied by mood swings and sleeping problems. A woman's vagina can become dry as secretions lessen and this can cause soreness. Sometimes a medicine such as clonidine hydrochloride (Dixarit) which is a beta-blocker and also prescribed for the prevention of migraine, can be given for menopausal flushing. Beta-blockers can prevent many of the physical manifestations of the tension that go with the menopause. They 'block' – stop – some of the unnecessary automatic nervous reactions to anxiety, such as a rapid heart beat. Feelings of insecurity and anxiety are common for some women with the menopause. Tampovagan pessaries, which contain oestrogen, can be given for menopausal vaginitis.

Symptoms of the menopause can be relieved by hormone replacement therapy – see page 93. Self-help measures include eating a well-balanced diet and taking exercise to help you relax. Get out in the open air – the body uses sunshine to make vitamin D which helps keep bones strong. Try to stop smoking – the menopause lowers the amount of oestrogen in your body and smoking increases this effect even more. Don't drink too much alcohol – in addition to being bad for the heart and liver, it can also lead to flushing and it's wise to limit alcohol intake to a reasonable level.

Preparations prescribed Dixarit, Tampovagan

MIGRAINE

Anyone who's ever had a migraine – and you can include me in that – can understand the misery it brings. Yet migraine sufferers are often branded as 'neurotic' and made to feel guilty about their 'weakness'. This is completely unfair, as studies have shown that there is not a typical 'migraine personality'. Migraine affects as many as one in ten people (mainly women) of any race, occupation, class or age, including children. More than half will have a relative – often their mother – with the same problem.

Frequency of attacks varies greatly, from only once or twice a year to several times a week. Severity and type of symptoms differ widely, too. A sufferer may find that he or she has a mild attack at one time and then a severe one next time. The severity is usually related to extra tension and strain and it is really very important to remain as calm as possible.

So what makes a migraine more than 'just a headache'? The pain is usually one sided, and in the 'common' type, there are other symptoms such as loss of appetite, nausea or vomiting. A few sufferers will have the 'classic' type of migraine, preceded, 20–30 minutes before the headache itself, by warning symptoms – called an aura – which may include flashing lights before the eyes, shimmering or double vision, slurred speech, numbness and giddiness. These symptoms are probably due to a sudden constriction in some of the blood vessels in the brain.

The headache comes on as these vessels then expand and the blood surges through, leading to the characteristic throbbing headache. Many experts believe that this constriction and dilation of the blood vessels is brought about by changing levels of certain chemicals circulating in the body, such as adrenaline – also released during stress – and prostaglandins. Adrenaline tenses the muscles, the heart and its blood vessels to prepare us for 'fight or flight'. Prostaglandins sensitise the nerve endings to make us more alert. In susceptible people, they will 'overdo' it and cause the above symptoms. Studies also suggest that there may be a slight difference – perhaps inherited – in the biochemical make-up of migraine sufferers which makes them more susceptible.

The trigger for an attack can be emotional or physical and common ones include anxiety, excitement, depression, changes in weather or routine, bending for long periods (such as when gardening), hot baths, loud noises, flashing or bright light, including that from a VDU screen. Glare filters are now available which many people find helpful. Alcohol, especially red wine, is one of the worst culprits, and certain foods for example chocolate, cheese, fried foods, citrus fruit, onions, tea, coffee, wheat flour, pork and seafood are other common triggers.

Irregular meals, dieting or a long lie-in can provoke a migraine, probably because of the drop in the body's blood sugar. Then a few biscuits or a sweet drink may be enough to stave off a full attack. It's extremely important to make sure you always eat properly and pay attention to your diet. If you think you'll have to go a long time without a proper meal, keep an emergency ration of a small snack with you.

Hormones can also play a part as far as women are concerned – some only have a migraine around the time of their menstrual period or if they are taking the contraceptive pill. Many find their migraines improve, or stop altogether, after the menopause.

To help you and your doctor pinpoint your special triggers, try to keep a diary, noting the day and time of your attacks, everything you eat and drink, meal times, daily activities, particular worries and, for women, the dates of your periods. If you think you are suffering from migraine or experience a migraine attack for the first time, consult your doctor for a proper diagnosis and advice on treatment. This will also reassure you that your migraines are not due to a tumour or to high blood pressure – two very common and usually quite unfounded fears.

Treatment will depend on the frequency of attacks and the apparent causes. Simply adjusting your habits may help considerably. Any medicines should be taken at the first sign of an attack, so always keep them handy. It usually helps to rest quietly in a darkened room in the early stages. During a migraine attack, the action of the gut slows down and painkillers may not be well absorbed. Some of the medicines available from your doctor speed up absorption as well as relieving the nausea and pain. Other drugs act by constricting the dilated blood vessels, but follow the instructions precisely as overuse can actually bring on a headache similar to migraine.

If migraine attacks are very frequent, your doctor may prescribe long-term preventive treatment, such as one of the drugs often used to control high blood pressure, a beta-blocker such as metoprolol tartrate (Betaloc). Such medicines have an effect upon the blood vessels. Migraine occurs as the arteries to the brain first 'close' and then open and beta-blockers have been found to dampen this process (see also HIGH BLOOD PRESSURE, page 88). Remember that migraine is different from other types of headache in that it's often accompanied or preceded by other symptoms already mentioned.

Anti-inflammatory medicines like aspirin and ibuprofen can prevent the release of prostaglandins and so are recommended for migraine – although paracetamol can help ease the pain of a headache, too. Other medicines can contain analgesics combined with buclizine hydrochloride or cyclizine hydrochloride – antihistamines to prevent vomiting and reduce nausea. Or you may be prescribed an inhaler like Medihaler Ergotamine which contains ergotamine tartrate for the rapid relief of migraine.

You may be prescribed a medicine such as Sanomigran, for example, which contains the antihistamine pizotifen (a drug related to some of the anti-depressants). The medicine is used to prevent migraine headaches or reduce the frequency and severity but should be taken regularly. The prophylactic effect is associated with its ability to modify the chemical changes that accompany a headache. Such medicine can make people drowsy, cause dizziness, sickness or cause an increase in appetite or weight gain.

Another prescription medicine is Imigran. These tablets contain sumatriptan, the first of a new group of medicines developed for the treatment of migraine. As the symptoms of migraine may be due to swollen blood vessels around the brain, medicines like Imigran probably work by reducing the size of these blood vessels and are called 5HT1 agonists. Most people taking this medicine seem to find that it causes no problems, but if any of the following side-effects occur you should check with your doctor: sudden wheeziness, fluttering or tightness in the chest; swelling of eyelids, face or lips; skin rash. These symptoms could mean that you are allergic to the medicine. More rare side-effects include tiredness, dizziness, flushing, feelings of tingling, warmth, heaviness, pressure, tightness or sometimes pain in different parts of the body, including the chest and throat, weakness, nausea or vomiting when not part of migraine attack. These are not usually very troublesome and pass off with time.

Anti-emetics can be prescribed, too, to help control nausea or vomiting, see page 115.

Sufferers usually work out which treatment suits them

best. If stress or anxiety seems to be the underlying cause of your migraine, relaxation exercises or hypnotherapy may be helpful. And trying 'alternative' treatments like acupuncture is something many people try if they find no joy through traditional methods of coping with migraine.

Period-time migraines often respond to treatment with the hormone progesterone. Recent research has shown that a daily dose of a humble plant called feverfew helps many people to control their migraine. Two or three leaves can be eaten in a sandwich sweetened with a little honey, and feverfew capsules and tablets are available from some chemists and health-food shops.

Preparations prescribed Betaloc, Beta Prograne, Blocadren, Buccastem, Cafergot, Cardinol, Deseril, Dixarit, Imigran, Inderal, Inderal LA/Half-Inderal LA, Lingraine, Lopresor, Lopresor SR, Medihaler Ergotamine, Midrid, Migraleve, Migravess, Migravess Forte, Migril, Paramax, Periactin, Sanomigran, Stemetil

MORNING-AFTER PILL

The morning-after pill, or post-coital contraception, (Schering PC4) contains the hormones levonorgestrel (a progestogen) and ethinyl-oestradiol (an oestrogen). It's used as an occasional emergency measure after unprotected sex or an accident such as a condom rupturing, to prevent implantation of the fertilised egg.

Two tablets are taken as soon as possible after sex – up to a maximum of 72 hours afterwards – and the remaining two tablets twelve hours after the first two.

Nausea and vomiting are common side-effects. Vomiting could reduce the efficacy of the morning-after pill if it occurs within about two hours after the ingestion of either dose of tablets, in which case your doctor may advise taking more pills.

The pattern of periods is often temporarily disturbed and breast discomfort and headaches can also develop.

Preparation prescribed Schering PC4.

MOUTH ULCERS

Mouth ulcers tend to be small lesions on the inside of the cheeks, on the tongue, or the roof of the mouth. They are something that everybody seems to suffer from at some stage. They're often called aphthous ulcers and have a pale grey base and a slightly raised yellowish edge, tinged with a narrow, inflamed border.

Some people find that ulcers hurt so unbearably that eating is impossible. Fortunately, for most they're just a temporary nuisance. They may be painful but they are harmless and should disappear of their own accord after a week or so.

Despite all the research that has been carried out, we still have no real idea what causes mouth ulcers. We do know, however, that a person is more likely to develop them if he or she is under stress, unwell, over-tired, depressed or suffering from any form of emotional upset. People in high-powered jobs, young mothers and toddlers with flu all seem to be prone to attacks. Many women find they suffer from mouth ulcers almost monthly, around the time of their period.

You may get symptoms of an impending ulcer hours before they appear. The mouth will become over-sensitive or you'll experience a burning or tingling sensation. Pretty soon, blisters with red margins appear in your mouth. When they erupt they produce small, round ulcers with greyish or dirty white centres, which are often extra sensitive to salty and acidic foods.

Mouth ulcers may clear up within a few days or take over a week to disappear. In most cases, no treatment is needed. But if the ulcer is particularly painful, an antiseptic mouthwash or pastilles or gel containing antiseptics or local anaesthetic, such as Bongela, can ease soreness. Carbenoxolone sodium (Bioplex) helps the healing of mild ulcers, or lozenges and pastes containing corticosteroids such as triamcinolone (Adcortyl for example) as well as anti-inflammatory agents and an analgesic such as benzydamine hydrochloride (Difflam). An antibacterial solution containing chlorhexidine gluconate (Corsodyl) is another option. A supplement of folic acid, one of the B vitamins, may help shorten an atttack or prevent another one occurring.

If any ulcer is abnormally large or lasts for more than two weeks, you should certainly consult your doctor. And if you find you're getting frequent attacks of ulcers, even though they heal quickly, it may well be worth taking a careful look at the way you live and trying to reduce any stress in your life. Find a method of regular relaxation – that might mean taking a form of gentle exercise or listening quietly to music. Another simple way to combat stress is to try to get more sleep!

Preparations prescribed Adcortyl, Bioplex, Bonjela, Corsodyl, Difflam,

MUSCULAR ACHES, PAINS, SPRAINS AND STRAINS

As more and more people are heeding advice to take regular exercise a few are bound to suffer a so-called soft tissue (as opposed to bone) injury at some time – strains, sprains or bruising, for example, to muscles, ligaments, tendons or the capsule (lining) of a joint. The elderly and those who have taken up or returned to a sport late in life are more at risk than the young and fit.

A strain is a slight tearing of a muscle or the tendon attaching it to a bone, usually caused by overstretching it, whereas a sprain is a tear in a joint capsule or its supportive ligaments, due to twisting or forcing the joint beyond its normal range of movement.

Other soft tissue problems include capsulitis (inflammation of a joint lining due to a twisting or jarring injury), bursitis (inflammation of the fluid-filled bursae that act as cushions at points of wear and tear) and epicondylitis (inflammation where muscle tendons join the bony points of the elbow). If pain and tenderness are on the outer point, epicondylitis is commonly known as tennis elbow, if on the inner side golfer's elbow, but any activity that overuses these tendons can cause the same symptoms – painting a ceiling or hammering, for example. The characteristic overuse of one particular movement of the arm, in particular, inflames the tendons that make the movement and are known as a tendonitis.

Another condition, often in the news these days, is tenosynovitis or repetitive strain injury (RSI) – painful inflammation of the tendon sheaths in the hands, wrists or arms, which can be very disabling. Typists, factory workers or anyone using repetitive movements for hours on end are particularly prone. Regular rest breaks and more varied work will help prevent RSI developing.

When a sprain or strain first occurs, chemicals are released into the damaged tissues – they include prostaglandins, which sensitise nerve endings and cause pain, inflammation and swelling. Treatment which prevents or cuts down the release of prostaglandins is therefore likely to be helpful. Medicines known as NSAIDs – non-steroidal anti-inflammatory drugs – such as aspirin and ibuprofen, act in this way and the sooner they can be given after an injury the better (see PAINKILLERS, page 121). Ibuprofen can be given in the form of a gel – studies show that it relieves the pain and other symptoms when rubbed directly into the injured area, without the risk of side-effects, nausea for example, that tablets may cause (see BACK PAIN, page 28).

Lasonil is another cream that can help soft tissue injuries. It contains heparinoid, an anti-inflammatory agent. Sometimes an anti-inflammatory injection – into the tender spot of a tennis elbow, for instance – will be advised if the pain is acute.

First-aid measures in the initial 48 hours after injury can be very helpful and speed recovery. Rest the injured part as much as possible and raise it to reduce swelling (support an injured arm in a sling, for example). An ice pack will reduce the initial bruising and swelling and will also relieve pain; contrary to popular belief, a hot bath can make matters worse at first, because it speeds up the flow of blood and increases swelling. Wrap the ice in a wet cloth or flannel to protect the skin from iceburn and frostbite and apply the pack to the injured part for ten minutes every few hours. A compression bandage such as tubigrip, worn continuously for at least two days, will help, too, but watch for numbness, tingling or the skin colour changing to white or blue – signs that the bandage is too tight.

Preparations prescribed Algesal, Clinoril, Clinoril 200, Cremalgin Balm, Diclomax Retard, Difflam Cream, Disalcid, Fortagesic, Intralgin, Lasonil, Mobiflex, Motrin, Movelat, Oruvail Gel, Pranoxen Continus, Robaxin, Surgam, Trancopal, Voltarol Emulgel

NAPPY RASH

All babies suffer from a red or sore bottom from time to time, however well you look after them. For the first couple of years or so of a child's life, the area of skin around his or her bottom is constantly in contact with – and so under attack from – urine and faeces. Nappy rash can take the form of just a few spots, or a more severe rash. It can be triggered by several factors, such as diarrhoea or rawness caused by urine that's irritating the skin inside a chafing nappy. Bacteria in the faeces can react with urine to produce ammonia – not very pleasant on tender, young skin. This type of contamination often encourages a fungus similar to the one that causes thrush.

To avoid nappy rash change your baby's nappy frequently and clean and dry his or her bottom and skin creases thoroughly. It's helpful to leave your baby without a nappy on as often as possible – air is a great benefit. Use a barrier cream – zinc and castor oil cream, for example – to protect the baby's skin from constant exposure to moisture. If you use terry towelling nappies, be careful to sterilise them properly as well as ensuring that they're well rinsed – traces of detergent can also be an irritant.

If the baby's bottom already shows signs of a rash, specially formulated nappy rash creams can soothe it, help fight infection or prevent moisture irritating the skin. If the rash doesn't seem to get any better after a week of this treatment, ask the advice of your doctor or health visitor.

For severe nappy rash when thrush is a factor, a cream such as Timodine may be prescribed. This contains nystatin, an antifungal agent, hydrocortisone, a corticosteroid to soothe inflammation and benzalkonium chloride, an antiseptic. Creams containing hydrocortisone should be used for a week at most.

Preparations prescribed Cetavlex, Conotrane, Hydrocal, Kamillosan, Morhulin, Morsep, Siopel, Sudocrem, Timodine, Tinaderm-M Cream, Unguentum Merck

NAUSEA AND VOMITING

Nausea and vomiting are very common symptoms – causes include travel sickness, early pregnancy, eating and drinking too much, gastric disorders and reaction to treatment with cancer drugs. Careful diagnosis therefore needs to be made for the reason why a person is suffering in this way before appropriate treatment and advice can be given.

Anti-emetics are usually used to treat this problem. They can be divided into domperidone (such as

Motilium), metoclopramide (such as Gastrobid Continus) and phenothiazines – prochlorperazine maleate (such as Buccastem). They suppress pro-emetic stimuli by blocking certain chemical receptors in the brain, known to trigger the vomiting reflex. Anticholinergic anti-emetics are often used to control travel sickness (see page 157). Antihistamines are also used particularly when the problem is due to Menière's syndrome (see page 162).

Side-effects of anti-emetics and antihistamines can include drowsiness, dizziness, restlessness, and headaches for example.

An anti-emetic such as ondansetron (Zofran) can be prescribed for medical treatments which cause nausea and vomiting. Side-effects are not common but can include sudden chest tightness or wheeziness, heart pounding, swelling of eyelids, face or lips, skin rash. Others include headache, feeling of 'warmness in the head or stomach', lightheadedness, flushes of the face, mild stomach cramps, upset bowels – constipation or diarrhoea. If you experience any of these, discuss them with your doctor as soon as possible.

Preparations prescribed Avomine, Buccastem, Dramamine, Gastrobid (when associated with stomach problems), Motilium, Phenergan, Stemetil, Stemetil Eff, Valoid, Zofran

ORAL THRUSH

Denture wearers may be familiar with the problem of oral thrush as a result of chafing, although it can also affect babies, people suffering from diabetes, those who are generally unwell and not at their strongest, or those taking steroid or antibiotic drugs.

It's caused by a yeast-like fungus called *candida albicans* which is also responsible for vaginal thrush. This fungus usually lives harmlessly in the mouth and intestines. Bacteria are normally able to keep it under control, but sometimes it will suddenly grow very rapidly, producing soreness and white flecks inside the mouth, painful cracks in the skin in the corners of the mouth and/or creamy yellow patches inside the mouth and throat.

If you think you or your baby have oral thrush, consult a doctor who may prescribe an antifungal medicine such as Daktarin Oral Gel, itraconazole (Sporanox) or lozenge such as Fungilin (amphotericin). Thrush will not go away without treatment. But if the patient is your baby, you can help by sterilising dummies frequently and, if you're breast feeding, taking extra care with nipple hygiene.

Preparations prescribed Daktarin Oral Gel, Fungilin, Sporanox

OSTEOPOROSIS

Osteoporosis, a thinning of the bones, is a painful condition that causes bones to become brittle so that they cannot withstand the wear and tear of everyday activities. They then break easily. Indeed, sufferers who fracture a hip often believe a fall has caused it when, in fact, it's more likely that the weight of the body alone was enough to bring about the fracture, which then caused them to trip and stumble.

Women after the menopause are particularly prone to thinning of the bones – as many as one in four women following the menopause is likely to develop osteoporosis compared with less than one in forty men of that age. Men have a denser bone structure than women, which makes them less at risk, but it may also be because they don't have the dramatic reduction of the hormone oestrogen that women undergo during the menopause. This hormone is particularly important in cases of osteoporosis because it helps the body to absorb the calcium it needs for the maintenance of strong, healthy bones.

If you're a woman, the older you are the more likely

you are to be affected by osteoporosis. Half of women over the age of seventy-five will develop osteoporosis. Small, fair, thin-boned women are particularly at risk, and unfortunately it does run in families because mothers and sisters are likely to be of similar build. Also prolonged use of some drugs such as steroids, anti-convulsants and antacids can lead to osteoporosis. Other factors that make it more likely include a late puberty or an early menopause, not having children, illnesses such as rheumatoid arthritis, hyperparathyroidism – when the thyroid gland overproduces its hormone, calcitonin – and asthma. Excessive smoking or drinking and not enough regular exercise can also be contributory.

There is a great deal of debate about the best methods of treatment. Calcium supplements should only be needed if your diet fails to provide you with enough. Treatments suggested have included calcium and fluoride tablets. Medicines include a preparation like Sandocal which contains calcium. This medicine is taken to slow down or stop calcium loss from bones in osteoporosis. It's also taken to treat calcium deficiency.

A few people can be upset by taking calcium supplements. Side-effects can include constipation, diarrhoea, nausea or vomiting, feeling very thirsty, passing water more frequently, anorexia, abdominal pain, bone pain, muscle weakness, drowsiness, confusion.

Other treatments are painkillers, anabolic steroids such as nandrolone decanoate (Deca-Durabolin) or thyroid hormones such as salcatonin (Calsynar), as well as physiotherapy and hydrotherapy in some cases.

But in my opinion, for most women, hormone replacement therapy (HRT, see page 93) begun at the time of the menopause and continued for at least ten years, is the most effective way to prevent osteoporosis. HRT provides the means of administering the female hormone oestrogen.

Most osteoporosis is thought to be preventable. If you're thinking of prevention, you need to be planning ten to twenty years ahead at least. Developing strong healthy bones depends partly on maintaining a good supply of calcium in our diet. This is particularly important during childhood, adolescence, pregnancy and while breastfeeding, and also the ten years before the menopause and for ten years after, when the body's absorption of calcium becomes less efficient due to hormonal changes.

Preparations prescribed Cacit, Calcisorb, Calsynar, Didronel PMO, Deca-Durabolin, Durabolin, Ossopan, Sandocal

PAINFUL OR HEAVY PERIODS

Seven out of ten women are thought to have painful periods (dysmenorrhoea) and three in ten women, heavy periods (menorrhagia). As if the pain isn't bad enough, some women experience sickness, vomiting, headache, fainting and diarrhoea as well.

When a young woman gets painful periods it's nearly always because the womb goes into spasm. Doctors call this primary dysmenorrhoea to distinguish it from secondary dysmenhorroea, the kind of period pain that mainly affects older women.

Secondary dysmenorrhoea can be caused by disorders such as endometriosis (when the womb-lining tissue develops outside the womb, see page 73), fibroids (benign tumours of the womb's muscular wall) or a continuing infection – pelvic inflammatory disease, for example.

In most cases painful periods are not a sign of ill health, but women who suddenly develop them should go to see their doctor, so that the cause can be treated appropriately. An ultrasound scan may occasionally be needed to detect – or rule out – any underlying disorder.

Sufferers from primary dysmenorrhoea sometimes have more of a chemical called prostaglandin in their menstrual flow than most women. The production of an egg, or ovum, in the middle of the month triggers the release of this excess prostaglandin, which sends pain signals to the brain – so when a woman doesn't ovulate she usually doesn't experience pain. That's why many women who suffer from painful periods are advised to take the contraceptive pill, which generally works by preventing ovulation. This is a relatively straightforward form of bringing relief.

Painkillers also help you cope with period pain. An anti-inflammatory one containing ibuprofen can inhibit the production of prostaglandin, which is why it can be so effective in relieving symptoms. Aspirin has the same effect. Mefenamic acid, which is an even more powerful prostaglandin dampener, has to be prescribed by your doctor. The most commonly prescribed medicine for period pain is Ponstan (mefenamic acid). Studies have indicated that it reduces the number and intensity of uterine contractions. As you should only need to take the drug for a few days at one go, this reduces the likelihood of side-effects (see PAINKILLERS page 121).

There are also antispasmodic medicines available on prescription. These will relieve symptoms by relaxing the uterine muscles. An example is Spasmonal (alverine citrate).

Menorrhagia – heavy or irregular periods – are probably due to an often mild derangement of the body's hormone control, though the symptom may be very distressing. Traditionally, benign growths of the uterus, known as fibroids, have been thought to be responsible. However, research gynaecologists now have reasons to think that they are not so much to blame as was previously thought. They can also be treated with Ponstan to help reduce blood flow. Danazol (Danol) can be given to control excessive blood loss and pain. It's also used to treat endometriosis. Your doctor may also advise you to go on the pill, or you may be given a non-contraceptive progestogen preparation such as Primolut-N or Menzol which contain norethisterone (see ENDOMETRIOSIS, page 73).

Anti-fibrinolytic drugs, which quieten the enzymes which dampen clot formation, such as Cyklokapron (tranexamic acid) can be useful. They can cause nausea, vomiting and diarrhoea but this usually settles down if the dose is lowered.

Hot baths and hot water can also be soothing for period pain. Heat can help reduce muscle spasm, as can brisk exercise such as cycling, swimming and fast walking. A good, well-balanced diet with enough vitamin B6 and other B vitamins is helpful too.

Once a woman has her first baby, the painful periods of the primary dysmenorrhoea kind will usually go for good.

Preparations prescribed Buscopan, Codafen, Cyklokapron, Danol, Dolobid, Dolobid 500, Duphaston, Menzol, Orudis, Ponstan, Pranoxen Continus, Primolut-N, Solpadol, Spasmonal

PAINKILLERS

Painkillers, or analgesics, can be used to treat pain resulting from a wide variety of symptoms. They can ease pain in headaches, migraine, neuralgia, colds and influenza and help reduce temperature, rheumatic pain, period pain, dental pain, back ache, muscular pain and sore throats.

There's a vast range of analgesics on sale in shops, supermarkets and chemists in soluble or tablet form. Soluble painkillers are said to work more quickly because the active ingredient is absorbed into the bloodstream faster than solid tablets. And there's also quite a choice at your doctor's disposal.

Analgesics contain aspirin, paracetamol or a combination of the two, sometimes with the addition of the stimulant caffeine. Some also contain small quantities of codeine and others contain ibuprofen. If you are taking one kind of analgesic you should not take another within four hours – overdoses can be dangerous.

Aspirin, and its associated sodium salicylate compounds, is a non-narcotic (non-addictive) analgesic. It relieves pain, reduces fever and inflammation, and can improve the symptoms of arthritis. It's also thought to prevent blood clots from forming. It works by blocking the production of prostaglandins, which would pass pain signals on to the brain.

Aspirin can irritate the stomach, and if it's used for a long time it can cause bleeding. That's why aspirin should be taken after food; if you must take it on an empty stomach, have a glass of milk at the same time. Avoid alcohol when you're taking aspirin, as it adds to the chances of the stomach being irritated. Do not take aspirin if you have a stomach ulcer. It is not usually recommended near the end of a pregnancy, either.

There also appears to be some connection between young children taking aspirin and developing Reye's Syndrome – a rare condition, affecting only about seven children in a million, which causes brain inflammation and liver damage. It is not even certain that aspirin is implicated in this condition, but the possibility is enough to make doctors feel that children under 12 should not generally be given aspirin. Paracetamol is a safe alternative.

Painkillers specially formulated for children usually include paracetamol and can be used for headache, migraine, neuralgia, toothache, pain in teething, sore throat, aches and pains, for the symptomatic relief of rheumatic aches and pains; influenza, feverishness and feverish colds and childhood infections such as chickenpox, whooping cough, measles and mumps; and for the symptomatic relief of reactions due to vaccination or immunisation. Side-effects from paracetamol administered in normal doses are rare.

Paracetamol is also a non-narcotic analgesic. It's gentler on the stomach than aspirin and won't cause bleeding. But large doses can cause serious damage to the liver and kidneys. It can be used during pregnancy, but always check with your doctor if you think you need to take it for more than an occasional dose.

Paracetamol works in a similar way to aspirin, but, unlike aspirin, it only blocks prostaglandin production in the brain, rather than elsewhere in the body as well. This means that it does not reduce inflammation, as aspirin does.

Ibuprofen is an NSAID (non-steroidal anti-inflammatory drug) which relieves pain, reduces inflammation and lowers temperature. It has been found in use to be gentler on the stomach than aspirin (though there is no obvious explanation for this as they work in similar ways) and as a result is almost as well tolerated as paracetamol. However, as with other pain-relievers, it shouldn't be taken if you have a stomach ulcer or other stomach disorder. Asthma sufferers and anyone who is allergic to aspirin should only take ibuprofen after consulting their doctor.

Other NSAIDs include mefenamic acid, indomethacin, diflusinal, ketoprofen and naproxen. This group of drugs is commonly prescribed for muscle and joint pain. They are also useful for period pain.

Codeine is a mild narcotic (habit-forming) drug used in combination with paracetamol, or paracetamol and aspirin. It blocks transmission of pain signals within the brain and the spinal cord, but used on its own does not have much painkilling effect. While its use in combination as mentioned above has always been popular, the benefits of this over the use of aspirin and paracetamol on their own are open to doubt. Do not take codeine-containing medicines if you are pregnant, or think you may be, as it has not been tested to prove that it is safe during pregnancy. However, do not be alarmed if you took a tablet or two before you knew you were pregnant, since it has not been specifically shown to cause any harm either.

Other narcotics include morphine, pethidine, phenazocine and methadone. These are usually used to control severe pain. Their use is strictly controlled since many are highly addictive and can readily become drugs of abuse. In general painkillers can cause a variety of side-effects, in particular constipation or nausea.

Preparations prescribed Acupan, Aloxiprin, Alvedon Suppositories, Aspav, Aspirin, Benoral, benorylate, Brufen, Calpol Infant, Caprin, co-codamol, co-codaprin, Codafen Continus Tablets, codeine phosphate (occasionally used alone although its effect is then limited), co-dydramol, co-proxamol, dextropropoxyphene, DHC Continus, dihydrocodeine, Disprol Paediatric, Dolobid, fenoprofen, Flexin Continus, LS and Flexin-25, Junifen, Nu-Seals aspirin, Orudis, Palaprin, Panadol, Panadol Extra/Suspension, paracetamol, Paramax, pentazocine, Progesic, Ponstan, Solpadol, Sevredol Tablets and Suppositories, Tylex

PARKINSON'S DISEASE

Many of the symptoms of Parkinson's Disease such as stiffness, bent stature, and a general slowing down can be mistaken for those of normal ageing. Also, the onset and progress of the disease tends to be gradual so the diagnosis may be missed for some time. However, Parkinson's disease is not just due to ageing although the chances of developing it do increase with age – one in every hundred men and women over sixty, but sometimes younger, will be affected. There is no real evidence that the condition is hereditary.

Some specialists believe that the degeneration of the nerve cells at the base of the brain that occurs in this disease may be caused by an, as yet unidentified, toxin in the environment to which some people are susceptible. These 'basal' nerve cells normally produce neurotransmitters – chemicals such as dopamine – necessary for relaying nerve impulses or 'messages' to the muscles via a complex system which is essential for most of the movements we take for granted.

In Parkinson's disease, these nerve cells slowly degenerate and fail to produce enough dopamine, leading in time to a wide range of possible symptoms. One of these is the typical tremor, often occuring in just one hand or arm, usually worse at rest and improving during activity. There are other causes of the 'shakes' such as 'benign essential tremor' but this common and relatively harmless condition tends to be absent at rest and worse when the arms are outstretched or active. Certain drugs, such as those given long-term for mental illness, are among other causes of tremor.

Someone with Parkinson's disease will probably find that their writing becomes progressively smaller and fine movements, such as tying shoelaces, are difficult. Balance is often affected and speech may be slow, monotonous and slurred – giving the false and embarrassing impression of being drunk. Another distressing symptom is loss of facial expression, making the sufferer appear not 'all there' although in fact the intellect is not affected.

Depression is also a common part of the illness and anti-depressant medicines can then be very helpful.

Treatment of Parkinson's disease has been revolutionised by the drug levodopa (Brocadopa, Madopar, for example) which is given as tablets and converted in the body to dopamine. This, prescribed in combination with other drugs, effectively replaces the natural dopamine that is lacking and reverses many of the distressing symptoms, often allowing the sufferer to continue their usual way of life. Side-effects can include nausea, vomiting and anorexia.

The benefits of levodopa may begin to wear off after several years but new drugs now being used as well, such as selegiline (Eldepryl), reduce this risk.

Selegiline is a medicine which inhibits a brain enzyme (called selective MAO-B, for short). This allows one of the body's natural chemical 'healers', dopamine, to act for longer and so helps to even out and prolong the effect of dopamine. This includes L-dopa, which is given as a medicine, as well as any natural dopamine that the sufferer's brain continues to produce.

Recent studies have shown that use of this drug in patients who have not been treated before can delay the development of disability and even prolong the time before they need to take levodopa. Side-effects seem to be isolated but can include hypotension and nausea. Muscle spasm and psychosis have also been reported.

Dopamine agonists which stimulate surviving dopamine receptors in the brain are also used. Examples include bromocriptine (Parlodel), or lisuride (Revanil). Amantadine (Symmetrel) can treat mild symptoms. Other drugs dampen certain chemical transmitters in the brain. Examples are orphenadrine (Disipal, Biorphen), benztropine (Cogentin), procyclidine (Kemadrin) methixene (Tremonil) among others.

The dose and combination of drugs that the doctor prescribes is tailored to the individual and constantly reassessed and balanced to achieve maximum benefit with minimum side-effects.

Regular exercise such as a daily walk is important whenever possible. Specific exercises from a physiotherapist will help prevent muscle weakness and maintain flexibility. Independence in daily tasks should also be encouraged. Speech therapy and occupational therapy, including advice on various aids, can be very helpful. The diet should contain plenty of roughage as constipation is often a problem.

Recently an experimental surgical treatment has hit the headlines. It involves transplanting dopamine-producing brain cells from a human aborted foetus into the Parkinson sufferer's brain but so far only a very few operations have been carried out and there are ethical problems. In some cases improvement in symptoms has occurred but it is not yet known whether any benefits will be lasting. Much more scientific evaluation is needed but the treatment holds out hope for the future.

Preparations prescribed Biorphen, Brocadopa Capsules, Broflex, Cogentin, Disipal, Eldepryl, Kemadrin, Madopar, Madopar Cr, Parlodel, Revanil, Symmetrel Capsules, Symmetrel Syrup, Tremonil.

PERENNIAL RHINITIS

Having a cold once or twice a year, as most of us do, is bad enough. Imagine what it would be like to have cold-like symptoms all the year round. Probably about one person in ten – children and adults – suffers in this way.

Rhinitis is simply an inflammation of the mucous membrane lining the nose and there are many possible causes. Seasonal rhinitis (see HAY FEVER, page 81) occurs as an allergic reaction to pollens and other allergens around at a particular time of year. In between while the symptoms disappear.

In the case of perennial rhinitis, however, the nose remains inflamed and unpleasant symptoms – which may include a constantly blocked or runny nose, itchy eyes and frequent sneezing – persist. The sense of taste and smell can also be affected and the sufferer often feels generally 'under the weather'. If he or she experiences these symptoms for more than one hour in 24 on most days of the year, a diagnosis of perennial rhinitis can be made. Children who suffer from perennial rhinitis typically develop a 'nose crease' from constantly rubbing their itchy nose upwards; nose bleeds are quite common and dark circles under the eyes may be another sign.

So what causes these continuing symptoms? In a few cases they will be due to a physical obstruction in the nose, such as polyps. Sometimes they will be a reaction to certain drugs, to changes in hormone levels – during pregnancy and at the menopause, for instance – or to changes in temperature or humidity. Irritating conditions at work, such as smoke or fumes, can also be responsible.

Most often, however, symptoms are due to an allergy – to animal fur and hair, for example, or to house dust mites which, invisible to the naked eye, exist in their millions in the furnishings, floors and bedding of even the cleanest home. The house dust mites lives on the dead skin cells that we shed constantly and each produces 40 faecal pellets a day – not a pretty thought! Fortunately, most of us co-exist quite happily with our house-dust mites, but these pellets are the trigger that provokes the allergic response and symptoms of perennial rhinitis in those susceptible.

Sufferers can minimise their problem by vacuuming floors and furnishings and damp-dusting frequently, covering mattresses with a plastic cover and using pillows and duvets made from artificial fibres rather than feathers. Polished boards or vinyl floor coverings are less of a mite-trap than carpets. Mites thrive in warmth, so keep the bedrooms cool and well aired. Smaller objects, such as children's fluffy toys, can be put into the deep freeze every so often – mites cannot survive at that temperature.

Many people who suffer from perennial rhinitis just put up with it – they think the symptoms are too trivial to bother their doctor with – or they try to treat themselves with medicines bought from the chemist, such as nasal decongestant sprays. Although these can be all right, used sparingly, for the short-term relief of the blocked nose at the end of a common cold, they are quite unsuitable for treating the long-term blocked nose of perennial rhinitis. Overuse of these sprays will soon damage the lining of the nose and actually make the condition worse with so-called 'rebound congestion'. Antihistamines bought over the counter will temporarily dry up a runny nose, but they will have no effect on a blocked nose and can cause drowsiness.

When nasal symptoms are persistent, it is important to consult a doctor, as there are several effective treatments that he or she can prescribe once the possible non-allergic causes already described have been excluded. Obviously, identifying the allergen so that the sufferer can avoid it as far as possible is helpful. Alternatively, anti-allergic, anti-inflammatory nasal sprays or drops, such as sodium cromoglycate (Rynacrom, for example) or corticosteroids, if used consistently as directed, are very effective at both preventing and relieving symptoms. Sufferers often have, or have had, other allergic-type conditions, such as eczema or asthma, or these may run in the family. Successful treatment of rhinitis can also keep asthma attacks at bay.

So it is well worthwhile consulting your doctor if you seem to have a permanent head cold or 'hay fever' – these always have a limited duration. Perennial rhinitis does not, but modern treatments will relieve it.

Preparations prescribed (see also HAY FEVER) Beconase Aqueous Nasal Spray, Beconase Nasal Spray, Flixonase Aqueous Nasal Spray, Rhinolast Nasal Spray, Rinatec, Rynacrom 4% Nasal Spray/Cartridges/Nasal Drops, Rynacrom Compound, Tavegil

PILES

Piles, or haemorrhoids, are actually enlarged, worn-out veins – varicose veins that may feel rather like soft, spongy grapes. They're found in and around the lower rectum and anal canal at the very lowest end of the bowel, in a pad of tissue that is not unlike the lips found at the opposite end of the digestive system! Nature intended this soft tissue to be there because, when healthy, it makes a very good seal. But when the veins within it enlarge, becoming piles, a discharge of mucus from the anus can be just one of many distressing symptoms.

Doctors believe that at least half the people in Britain suffer from piles at some time in their life, although many are too embarrassed to seek advice. A susceptibility seems to run in families, perhaps due to an inherited weakness in the wall of the rectal blood vessels. The veins the walls contain, unlike veins elsewhere, do not have valves in them to aid the flow of blood. If anything increases the pressure on these rectal veins, they can become engorged and distended, just like varicose veins in the leg. So there is really no need to be embarrassed about having piles – the chances are that the doctor or pharmacist you consult will have had them too! They really are very common, even more so in men than in women. You are more likely to suffer from piles as you get older (especially if you are overweight), although quite young people can be troubled by them too.

There are many old wives' tales about the causes of piles. Despite popular belief, you do not get them by sitting on cold walls or hot radiators. Perhaps surprisingly, active sportsmen and women are prone to piles and, like varicose veins, they are a particular hazard of pregnancy. The weight of the developing baby can put pressure on the rectal veins, causing them to enlarge as the normal flow of blood is prevented. Fortunately, these piles usually subside after the baby's birth and treatment meanwhile can relieve the discomfort.

Some medicines, such as codeine and iron tablets, if taken regularly, can be constipating and so predispose to piles. Chronic constipation, with the straining and increased pressure on the veins this brings, is one of the most common causes, as is a lack of fibre in the diet over many years.

If you have piles, the first sign you may notice is some bright red blood in the lavatory, or on the loo paper, after a bowel movement. It is always important to check with your doctor that this bleeding is caused by piles and not by some other condition.

'Internal' piles – also known as 'first degree' piles – which remain inside the anus are usually painless, but as the normal seal there is affected by the swollen veins, a constant, sometimes blood-stained, discharge may occur. There may also be itching and an uncomfortable feeling.

Second degree, 'external' piles, which prolapse through the anus, particularly when a motion is passed, tend to become inflamed, itchy and painful from time to time. They usually slip back, or can be gently pushed back, in between bowel movements. It may be easiest to do this while having a bath or using a bidet, when the area is lubricated with soap and your hands are clean.

If second degree piles are not treated, they may protrude permanently – when they are known as third degree piles – and cause considerable discomfort. Occasionally, a protruding pile will be gripped by the tight muscular band (sphincter) at the exit to the anus and become strangulated, which is very painful. If the blood inside the pile then clots, it will, in time, drop off – providing Nature's cure. Otherwise, rest in bed with the foot of the bed raised and an ice pack applied to the pile should relieve acute symptoms.

Less severe piles can often be cured completely by avoiding constipation and straining. So, if you have ever suffered from piles, or think you are likely to because they run in your family, do all you can to avoid becoming constipated. This means eating plenty of high-fibre foods – fresh fruit and vegetables, wholemeal bread and bran cereals, for instance. Fibre-containing tablets or drinks, such as Fybogel or Regulan, available from your chemist, can be helpful if you find it difficult to eat enough bran-type foods. Try also to cut down on salt and have plenty of watery or fruit drinks. This type of diet should keep your motions regular, well-formed and effortless. Laxatives are usually only advisable as a short-term measure.

If your symptoms persist, you may be prescribed some suppositories and/or ointments. These mainly contain local anaesthetics such as lignocaine or cinchocaine with a steroid (such as Proctosedyl hydrocortisone and cinchocaine hydrochloride) to ease irritation, and astringents, bismuth subgallate for example (Anusol), to help dry up piles and relieve inflammation. A cream such as Betnovate rectal ointment which contains betamethasone valerate (also a topical steroid) with lignocaine to reduce pain and itchiness and phenylephrine (a vasoconstrictor) will help reduce any swelling.

If your piles keep recurring and being troublesome, your doctor will probably refer you to a surgeon for further advice. A suppository is usually inserted after each bowel movement and at night and in the morning. Suppositories should never be taken orally. Some are said to be safe to use in pregnancy, but always check this with your pharmacist. Injection treatment may be recommended for bleeding internal or less severe external piles. This involves injecting a special fluid into the dilated veins which causes them to shrink. You will be treated as an outpatient and although the procedure may sound unpleasant, it is not painful and is usually very successful. In fact, it's one of the easiest and quickest forms of treatment.

As an alternative, cryosurgery – 'freezing' the veins – may be used, or constricting bands may be placed around the base of the veins. An operation under general anaesthetic, called 'Lord's procedure' can be very effective even for quite advanced piles. It involves a powerful stretching of the tight sphincter muscles around the anus. For severe third degree piles, however, many surgeons will advise removing them completely. This operation may cause discomfort for some time afterwards, but it should then solve the problem once and for all.

Preparations prescribed Anacal, Anugesic-HC, Anusol, Anusol HC, Betnovate Rectal Ointment, Carbalax, Proctosedyl, Scheriproct Ointment and Suppositories, Ultraproct Ointment and Suppositories, Xyloproct Ointment, Xyloproct Suppositories

PILL, THE

The contraceptive pill has been the subject of more publicity and controversy than probably any other medicine. This is partly because, unlike other medicines, it is taken not to cure or relieve symptoms but by healthy women, so any risk involved is more unacceptable. However, many people choose to continue smoking in spite of the known, far greater, risks and widely-used medicines, such as aspirin, are also potentially far more harmful than the pill. Take an overdose of the pill and you will come to no lasting harm, whereas an overdose of aspirin could be fatal.

Although undoubtedly the pill is not suitable for all women, the ultra low-dose pills now available and the tri-phasic pills (the dosage in these is related to the natural ebb and flow of the woman's hormones) have helped reduce any risks and side-effects to a minimum. Studies done over the 30 years since the pill has been in use have also given doctors clearer and safer guidelines for prescribing it so that women at any particular risk can be singled out and an alternative method of contraception advised. For millions of women, however, the pill continues to be a simple, reversible and virtually 100% effective method for which they are thankful.

There are two main types of pill, the most commonly-used combined pill (which contains a combination of the two hormones oestrogen and progestogen) and the so called 'mini-pill'. This is not, as some people believe, just a low-dose combined pill, but is different altogether as it contains only one hormone – progestogen – and acts in quite a different way to prevent conception. When taking the combined pill, the circulating hormones normally 'trick' the body into thinking it has already ovulated. The ovaries do not therefore receive their usual 'message' to release an egg – so, no egg, no pregnancy. On those occasions when ovulation does occur, the pill's other effects upon the lining of the womb prevent a pregnancy from occurring.

The mini-pill may also prevent ovulation but its main effect is to alter the consistency of the mucus around the cervix (the entrance to the womb) making it thick and impenetrable to the sperm. It acts, in other words, as a kind of barrier method. For the mucus to maintain this impenetrable consistency, it is important to take this type of pill about the same time each day. It is then only slightly less effective than the combined pill and may be recommended for breast-feeding mothers and others for whom the combined pill is contra-indicated – those over 35 for example.

Until recently, when a woman reached the age of 35, doctors would advise her against taking the 'combined' contraceptive pill – which contains the two hormones oestrogen and progestogen. An alternative sometimes suggested was the progestogen-only mini-pill but because this can make the periods irregular, or stop them altogether, anxiety about possible pregnancy is often a problem. So the choices available to the older couple, if they wished to avoid pregnancy until the menopause, were limited.

Although a woman's fertility starts to decline after about thirty and her hormones – which stimulate ovulation – do vary considerably in the ten years or so before her final period, a reliable method of contraception is essential during this time if a baby is not desired. A recent survey shows that, for couples in their thirties, sterilisation is now the most popular choice of contraception in the UK whereas before this age the pill was easily top of the league. For suitable women, the pill has many advantages over other methods – reliability, convenience and regular, pain-free, light 'periods' for example – and now the good news is that only those who smoke, are overweight or have other relative contra-indications, such as high blood pressure, need stop the pill at 35.

A new pill is now available specially formulated for women over thirty. Called Mercilon, it contains only 20 micrograms of oestrogen – a third less than the usual 30 mcgm pills. The combination with a new type of progestogen (desogestrel), carefully balanced, enables it to be just as effective as other pills. It is recommended for older women as their particular menstrual cycles are usually well regulated even by this low level of oestrogen which also has health advantages. Studies show that desogestrel benefits the skin and also appears to have a favourable effect on some of the risk factors associated with heart disease and strokes. The smaller dose of oestrogen in Mercilon means that some common side-effects of the usual pills – breast tenderness and nausea for example – are less likely. So this new pill could be a good choice if you are thirty or more and considering starting the pill or returning to it after a break. If, however, you are happily settled on another type of low-dose pill, discuss it with your doctor but there should be no need to change.

Unfortunately, the health risks of the pill have been more publicised than the health benefits and figures show that 91% of women in the older age group think that the pill is unsafe for them. In fact, research has proved that it actually protects against cancer of the womb and the ovaries, makes fibroids less likely, prevents vaginal dryness (and so can improve sex life), controls symptoms, such as hot flushes, in the years leading up to the menopause and prevents osteoporosis – thinning of the bones. As a result of these findings, family planning experts now advise that, as long as a woman is fit, there is no reason why she should not enjoy these benefits until the age of 45 or even until the menopause. The trend towards a healthier lifestyle – improved eating habits, regular exercise and no smoking – is now making more and more women suitable for the pill.

Full discussion with your doctor, and health screening checks such as regular cervical smears and blood pressure checks are needed before deciding whether, or for how long, the pill is right for you. However, with the low-dose ones now available and the reassuring evidence of their safety, it certainly could be.

Occasional side-effects of the combined pill include nausea, vomiting, headaches, breast tension, changed body weight or libido, depressive moods and chloasma – a browning of the face, also known as a pregnancy mask, which it resembles.

Side-effects of the mini pill include irregular bleeding, breast discomfort, headache or acne. In isolated cases there may be nausea, vomiting, dizziness, headaches, migraine, depressive moods, disturbances of appetite, allergic reactions.

Preparations prescribed Combined: Brevinor, Conova 30, Cilest, Eugynon 30, Femodene, Femodene ED, Loestrin 20,30, Marvelon, Mercilon, Microgynon 30, Minulet, Neocon 1/35, Norimin, Norinyl-1, Ortho-Novin 1/50, Ovran, Ovran 30, Ovranette, Ovysmen Biphasic and Triphasic BiNovum, Logynon, Logynon Ed, Synphase, Triadene, Tri-Minulet, Trinordiol, TriNovum, Trinovum Ed. Progestogen only: Femulen, Micronor, Microval, Neogest, Noriday, Norgeston

POST-NATAL DEPRESSION (PND)

Many mothers will remember feeling 'weepy' about three or four days after their baby's arrival. This is very common and is probably due to sudden changes in the mother's hormone levels – particularly the fall in progesterone – which occurs following childbirth. However, about one in ten mothers will develop a more severe type of post-natal depression either continuing on from the early 'blues' or starting within six weeks of leaving hospital or, occasionally, later still.

A mother suffering from PND will become increasingly miserable, tearful and unable to cope with everyday things she previously managed quite easily, leaving her feeling guilty and inadequate. She may be excessively worried about her own health or the baby's, lose interest in her looks, be frightened of meeting people and will often find it difficult to concentrate on anything.

It is easy to blame the exhaustion she feels on the demands of having a new baby but with PND the exhaustion – both mental and physical – is more extreme than normal tiredness. Sleep problems – either sleeping too much or too little – are common. Usually the depressed mother will have no interest in sex which can throw a great strain on the marriage if the husband does not understand that this is part of the illness. Moodiness and bad temper are other common symptoms which can adversely affect the whole family. Some women have obsessional thoughts about harming themselves or others, especially the baby, and it is then vital for them to confide in someone who can help. Very occasionally a much more severe form of post-natal depression develops, called puerperal psychosis, when symptoms become extreme, suicide a real possibility and admission to hospital is necessary.

It's thought that there could be a link between mood changes after labour and the dramatic reduction in progesterone which occurs at delivery, but it seems more likely that abnormal reactions to the hormone changes, rather than the changes themselves, are the cause of mood swings in some women.

A mother who has had PND once is at risk of having it again. So, following any subsequent births, it is wise to watch carefully for early symptoms of depression so that treatment can be prescribed to prevent it developing. Other risk factors include having had a previous bereavement, including a stillbirth, extreme anxiety during pregnancy, having no one to confide in, and an unhappy marriage. There are links between premenstrual syndrome and PND and it is quite common for the depression to become worse just before a period, and when breastfeeding is stopped. The contraceptive pill can make some women feel depressed, so it is usually advisable for a mother with PND to use another reliable method of birth control.

Having a new baby is supposed to be an exciting, happy time and most mothers are overcome with guilt if they cannot feel joyful. So, what can be done to help if PND is suspected? It is important for the mother to understand she has an illness which can be treated and to consult a doctor early on without feeling ashamed. Stress to her that this type of depression is only temporary and that treatment will always bring about a complete recovery. Cyclogest (progesterone) is a preventive treatment for women who have previously suffered from post-natal depression, to avoid recurrence. These pessaries (suitable for vaginal or rectal insertion) are prescribed in order to give a gradual reduction in progesterone levels until periods recommence. Side-effects can include periods occurring earlier than expected or more rarely, later. Soreness, diarrhoea and flatulence can happen with rectal administration.

Anti-depressant medicines are also effective and can be taken as long as is necessary without concern because, unlike tranquillisers, they are not addictive. Improvement is usually gradual so be patient but tell your doctor if you are not feeling better after about three weeks as he will probably want to try a different tablet or alter the dosage. Don't worry if he advises staying on anti-depressants for several months and then cutting down gradually – you may get a relapse if you stop them too suddenly or too soon.

Preparation prescribed Cyclogest

PREMENSTRUAL SYNDROME

Premenstrual tension (PMT) is increasingly becoming known as premenstrual syndrome. The word 'syndrome' is more accurate, because there are so many different symptoms associated with the changes before a period, not just the well-documented feelings of tension.

Premenstrual syndrome is a complex set of many different symptoms, both physical and emotional, which occur only in the two weeks before menstruation. Because of the wide range of these symptoms, from migraine to constipation, anxiety or just tiredness, many doctors in the past have not recognised PMS, and women have inappropriately been put on tranquillisers.

PMS is due to a hormonal imbalance which takes place regularly each month as the body adjusts itself in readiness for menstruation. Unlike men, whose hormone levels are constant, women's hormone levels change constantly throughout their reproductive lives.

PMS can start right from the first period, or when there's been a gap between periods, during the vast hormonal changes after pregnancy, following artificial changes in the hormonal balance with the pill, or sterilisation (although it shouldn't, scientifically) or if your periods have stopped due to an illness.

For many women one of the most distressing and frightening symptoms is loss of control over their feelings. Otherwise gentle women have become violent towards their children and partners. Some, totally out of character, have even committed crimes while suffering, particularly shoplifting.

There is no 'cure' for PMS but there is now a variety of possible treatments which either treat individual symptoms – sometimes diuretics, used temporarily, for the feelings of bloatedness associated with water retention – or which help reduce the hormonal imbalances that lead to all sorts of unpleasant symptoms.

Pessaries containing progesterone (Cyclogest, for example) can be prescribed. These are suitable for vaginal or rectal insertion, usually beginning on the 14th day of the menstrual cycle and continuing treatment until onset of menstruation. If you use barrier methods of contraception then the pessaries should be inserted rectally. Sometimes periods can start earlier than expected as a result of this treatment – or, more rarely, they may be delayed. Soreness, diarrhoea and flatulence can occur with rectal administration.

Tablets such as Menzol or Primolut N (norethisterone) for example, can ease premenstrual symptoms such as headache, migraine, breast discomfort, water retention, tachycardia and psychological disturbances. Take a tablet two to three times a day from the 19th to the 26th day of the cycle. Treatment should be repeated for several cycles. When treatment is stopped, you may find you remain symptom-free for a number of months. Side-effects of this type of treatment are not that frequent at standard doses – the commonest being breakthrough bleeding, particularly when treatment is continuous over a long period. Other reported effects include nausea, vomiting, acne, oedema, weight gain, headache and depression.

Many women find that evening primrose oil is helpful in treating premenstrual breast pain (cyclical mastalgia) as well as non-cyclical mastalgia. Efamast (gamolenic acid provided by evening primrose oil) may be prescribed. Gamolenic acid (GLA) is normally formed within the body from the dietary polyunsaturated fatty acid, linoleic acid. Patients with mastalgia have been reported to have lower than normal levels of GLA and its metabolites. Polyunsaturated fatty acids can modulate the binding of steroid hormones to their receptors. Therefore, low levels of GLA and its metabolites may lead to exaggerated peripheral effects of normal concentrations of ovarian hormones. This means that the body's own natural hormones will be able to do their usual job better. Administration of Efamast raises the blood levels of GLA and substances derived from it. Also, pyridoxine, vitamin B6, has been demonstrated to be effective in dealing with premenstrual syndrome.

Preparations prescribed Cyclogest, Duphaston, Efamast, Menzol, Primolut N

PRICKLY HEAT

Prickly heat is an extremely irritating skin rash which develops in hot weather. It occurs – more in some people than in others – when the small blood vessels under the skin widen as the temperature rises. The extra blood they then supply to the surface of the body acts as the body's radiator, allowing heat to escape, and the extra blood supplies the extra liquid which the sweat glands release as sweat. As the tissues swell with extra blood and tissue fluids, the skin becomes congested and the pores are squeezed and then blocked. The sweat builds up under the skin and causes a rash known as prickly heat or *miliaria rubra*.

Sufferers from prickly heat will quickly recognise the emergence of small red pimples or blisters. The tissues look red because the small blood vessels are open wide, while the engorged tissues cause discomfort and feel prickly.

There's no simple, quick remedy, but if you can immerse yourself in water to keep cool, you should feel better. Covering yourself with light, white clothing will help and, obviously, keeping out of direct sunlight is a good idea, too. Calamine cream or lotions will cool the skin and antihistamine tablets can bring great relief (see HAY FEVER page 81). Your favourite antihistamine tablet or one recommended by the pharmacist is what I would advise.

PSORIASIS

See DRY SKIN CONDITIONS page 66

RINGWORM

Despite its name, ringworm is a fungal skin infection, and has nothing to do with worms. Ringworm infection looks like ring-shaped, red, scaly or blistery patches that form on the skin. Although without knowing it, we all come into frequent contact with the spores – or seeds – of the fungi that cause ringworm, either as they float about in the air, or as we touch others who have them, remarkably few of us become afflicted. Fortunately, the same is true of many other germs with which we come into almost daily contact.

It's also remarkable that, with ringworm – like athlete's foot, which is caused by the same family of fungi – several members of the same household can share the same bathroom, or even the same bed, without catching the disease, in spite of its obviously infectious nature. Nobody knows quite why, although we do know that we all vary considerably in our susceptibility to most diseases.

Until the introduction of effective anti-fungal medicines over the past 50 years, ringworm used to be a real scourge for many sufferers. It would often cause a person's hair to fall out, leaving the scalp covered in unpleasant sores.

In the old days drastic measures, like a course of x-rays, were taken to try to 'sterilise' the skin. Such x-rays, however, had disastrous results in later years since at the time, the full force of their effects when directed at the skin weren't really known. They certainly cured the ringworm – though, in retrospect, it was like using a sledgehammer to crack a nut, since the powerful x-ray could cause growths which would appear years later on the affected skin.

Nowadays, following your doctor's recommended course of treatment is probably the best advice for curing ringworm. With today's effective anti-fungal preparations, the skin will eventually clear. Examples of medicines used are Masnoderm Cream containing the antifungal agent clotrimazole, Lamisil tablets (containing terbinafine, an allylamine antifungal) used when oral therapy is considered appropriate due to the site, severity or extent of the infection. Fulcin which contains griseofulvin, an antifungal antibiotic, can also be prescribed.

However, if you remain in conditions that encourage the fungus to grow, then it can return, even when anti-fungal antibiotics have been given by mouth. Once the antibiotic effect wears off, the fungus may return anyway, regardless of the conditions you are in, although after each treated attack, this becomes much less likely and should cease altogether when the passing of time is accompanied by a gradual build-up of the body's resistance.

Athlete's foot (see page 27) is another example of a fungus infection of the skin. The nails, too, can become infected with a skin fungus. They are particularly difficult to treat since the tough nail plate itself is not supplied with blood and is almost impermeable to liquids. Consequently, neither the body's antibodies nor antibiotics can penetrate the nail to destroy the fungus.

Preparations prescribed Fulcin Tablets/Oral Suspension, Lamisil, Loceryl, Lotriderm, Masnoderm Cream, Nizoral, Sporanox, Tineafax Cream, Trosyl Nail Solution

SCABIES

Itch mites, technically known as *sarcoptes scabei*, can cause intense irritation to the skin, and the owner. It's caused by a female mite burrowing into the skin so that she can lay eggs. Scabies is a condition that's spread by direct contact between children, sexual partners and often throughout a family home. It's treated by scabicidal drugs which kill the mites, such as monosulfiram (Tetmosol) which is used for treatment and prevention. The solution needs to be diluted with two to three parts water. Then your body needs to be washed carefully with soap and water and thoroughly dried. Apart from the face and scalp, the entire body should be painted with the dilute solution, which is rubbed well in and left to dry. This should take about ten minutes after which you can put your clothes back on. Very rarely this type of treatment causes a rash.

Malathion (Derbac-M for example) can also be used to

get rid of scabies or lindane (Quellada) or the older type of treatment benzyl benzoate (Ascabiol).

Try not to scratch. This can lead to the skin becoming infected, making the condition even more unpleasant for the sufferer. Infected skin lesions can be treated with Polyfax ointment, a topical antibacterial agent containing polymoxin B sulphate and zinc bacitracin.

Preparations prescribed Ascabiol, Derbac-M, Eurax, Lyclear Dermal Cream, Polyfax Ointment, Prioderm, Quellada, Tetmosol Soap, Tetmosol Solution

SHINGLES

Shingles is a rash of blisters on the skin accompanied by a severe stinging pain, caused by a virus – the *varicella zoster* virus – which is also responsible for chickenpox. Anyone who develops shingles will have had chickenpox in the past, sometimes without realising it, as one can have what is known as a 'subclinical' attack, in which no spots appear.

Antibodies to the virus develop in the bloodstream at the first infection and prevent further attacks of chickenpox. However, the virus is able to settle and lie dormant in a non-infectious state, in the 'junction boxes' of nerves supplying a part of the skin or – less commonly – muscles. Often it will cause no further trouble, but if it does, the result will be shingles.

All manner of events can trigger an attack. If you're emotionally or physically exhausted, or suffering from illness or injury – indeed, if your body's defences are not at their best for whatever reason – the virus can become active. The older you get, the more likely you are to develop shingles. Of those who reach their eighties at least one in two will have suffered.

The first symptom is usually pain over the area of skin supplied by the nerves harbouring the virus. The most common place is around the side of the body, along a line following a rib. It can occur on both sides of the chest, but it is an old wives' tale that if it meets in the middle the outcome is fatal – that just isn't true.

To have the best chance of success any treatment should be given early on, preferably at the painful stage which can be when, or just before, the blisters appear.

Your doctor will sometimes prescribe a course of tablets which may help to lessen and shorten the attack. Acyclovir (Zovirax Shingles Treatment pack) is often prescribed. This type of treatment can sometimes cause a skin rash. Antiviral applications to the affected area of skin can help, idoxuridine, for example (Herpid) and anaesthetic ointments or over-the-counter ointments containing calamine can also be soothing.

The surrounding skin should be kept clean to prevent other germs infecting the blisters, as this could interfere with healing and lead to scarring. Antibiotics may be needed if infection does occur.

Preparations prescribed Herpid, Symmetrel Capsules/ Syrup, Virudox, Xylocaine Ointment, Zovirax Shingles Treatment Pack

SINUS PAIN, NASAL CONGESTION AND CATARRH

See COLD, THE COMMON page 37

SLEEPLESSNESS

Sleep has been the subject of a great deal of research and the results, for insomniacs, are reassuring. It seems that, in the long run, Nature ensures that we get the sleep we need and there is no hard and fast rule on how much we should have – individuals differ considerably in this. What matters most is how you feel the next day – if you are alert and efficient, although you have had only five hours sleep, that was enough for you and comparisons with friends can cause unnecessary worry. Remember, too, that the need for sleep lessens as we grow older.

It is also reassuring to know that even a prolonged period of unsatisfactory sleep will do no serious harm, although you may feel a bit tired and irritable and be less efficient than usual. Eventually the body will catch up on its sleep debt. Experiments have shown that poor sleepers in fact often sleep more than they think they do, although perhaps not as deeply as others.

During sleep, children grow and the body's worn-out tissues are renewed. Sleep is needed to relieve mental fatigue more than physical fatigue – just resting in bed will do this.

It is not yet known whether the sleep induced by sleeping pills is as restorative as natural sleep. Sleeping pills (hypnotics) can be useful when taken for a short time, to re-establish a pattern of sleep after a crisis, say, or to relieve anxiety about not sleeping. But dependency can easily develop and can be difficult to break. A 'rebound' insomnia is also common after stopping the pills, making it very tempting to take them again.

Benzodiazapines should be used to treat insomnia only when it is severe, disabling, or subjecting the individual to extreme distress. An underlying cause for insomnia should be sought before deciding upon the use of benzodiazepines for symptomatic relief. Common adverse effects include drowsiness, sedation, blurring of vision, unsteadiness and ataxia.

Lorazepam, for instance, should only be used for the short-term treatment of insomnia associated with anxiety. Nitrazepam, for instance, should only be used for the short-term treatment of insomnia when it's severe or disabling.

Antihistamines with sedative/calming effects such as promethazine hydrochloride (Phenergan, Sominex, for example) can be given. Such preparations can cause drowsiness, dizziness, restlessness, headaches, nightmares, tiredness and disorientation in a few patients.

Another type of medicine zopiclone (Zimovane) may be used for insomnia that is debilitating or is causing severe distress. A mild bitter or metallic after-taste is the most frequently reported adverse effect. An alternative is a sedative medicine such as chloral hydrate (Noctec, Welldorm) which can cause gastric irritation, abdominal distension and flatulence.

A barbiturate such as amylobarbitone (Amytal) used to be widely prescribed, but rarely is now. Common side-effects include drowsiness, sedation, ataxia and vertigo. Barbiturates were found to be addictive and became widely used as drugs of abuse. Also, the barbiturates were far more dangerous if taken in relatively small overdosage than the more modern medicines precribed for short-term sleeping problems.

Elderly people will often ask their doctor for sleeping pills just because they find lying awake boring and feel they should be asleep, not because they are suffering any ill effects. However, fitful sleep is usual as we grow older and sleeping pills may cause confusion and make falls more likely.

Nearly everyone has times when they sleep badly – a hectic day at work, a difficult time with the children, problems of all kinds leave us feeling worked up or on edge, and make it hard to relax. But for a few, sleep is a lasting problem. They may find it difficult to fall asleep, or they may wake up frequently or very early. Twice as many women suffer as men, especially those with an anxious personality.

Depression is a common cause of sleeplessness and, if severe, both can be relieved by antidepressants. Pain – from arthritis for example – can interfere with sleep; so too can breathing difficulties and some medicines. Alcohol, tea, coffee and cigarettes are all stimulants, so should be avoided before going to bed, whereas a light snack or a milky drink can help induce sleep. A warm bath before going to bed can be very relaxing. And a good read in bed will eventually lead to drowsiness.

As other aids to better sleep, establish a regular routine of meal times, of getting up early and of going to bed at about the same time every night. This helps the body's 'internal clock'. Make sure your bed is comfortable and the room warm, but not too warm. Imagine a peaceful scene and concentrate on relaxing each part of your body in turn. Some daily exercise in the fresh air will make sound sleep more likely and talking over any problems with a sympathetic person can relieve one cause of insomnia – worry.

If night sweats during the menopause disturb your sleep, hormone replacement therapy (see page 93) can help. If noise is a problem, try ear plugs. Overweight people tend to sleep better and losing weight can mean losing sleep – but obviously it's best to get the balance right here!

Preparations prescribed Amytal, loprazolam, loraxepam, lormetazepam, nitrazepam, Noctec, Nytol, oxazepam, Phenergan, Sominex, Soneryl, temazepam, Trancopal, Welldorm, Zimovane

SORE NIPPLES

Breastfeeding can sometimes result in painful nipples. The most common cause is incorrect positioning. You should always make sure that your baby is sucking the whole darker ring around your nipple, called the areola, rather than just the nipple itself.

There's no need to keep washing your nipples – just follow your usual washing routine, but don't use soap on your nipples as this could irritate them. Keeping your nipples dry by exposing them to the air now and again helps, as does changing breast pads frequently. Some women find that allowing a little breast milk to dry on them after each feed is useful. A little Kamillosan applied to the nipple area will also relieve soreness.

Preparations prescribed Kamillosan, Morsep, Xylocaine Ointment

SORE THROAT

A sore throat is an infection which makes the throat red and sore; it is most often due to a viral infection which clears up by itself after three or four days. Pain can be relieved by taking soluble aspirin or your preferred painkiller. Avoid smoking if your throat is very sore. Mouthwashes containing an antiseptic, povidone-iodine for example (Betadine) may be helpful, or an analgesic and anti-inflammatory rinse containing benzydamine hydrochloride (Difflam) can help. Disinfectant lozenges containing benzalkonium chloride (Bradosol), antiseptic lozenges containing cetylpyridinium chloride (Merocet) or Merocaine which has a local anaesthetic, benzocaine, added may be soothing.

The exact cause of a sore throat can only be established as other symptoms develop. And there are many possible causes – it may be due to a virus and be the start of a cold or flu. It is also one of the first signs of German measles, pharyngitis or tonsillitis – the latter two of which may need antibiotics. So if sore throat symptoms persist, consult your doctor.

Preparations prescribed Betadine, Bradosol, Difflam Oral Rinse, Merocet, Merocaine, Tyrozets

STEROIDS

Steroids are near-relatives of many of the natural hormones produced in our body. For instance, our adrenal glands secrete them when we're injured or under stress and these hormones are natural, cortisone-type healing and calming agents. Other steroids are secreted internally to control the body's sexual functions.

The steroids that are prescribed to dampen down the inflammation of rheumatoid arthritis are of the cortisone type. Those taken – unofficially – by some sportspeople are called anabolic steroids and can cause a temporary increase in the mass and tone of the muscles of the body, as well as the speed with which the muscles work.

When used to relieve rheumatoid arthritis, steroids can be life-saving. Anabolic steroids for the treatment of muscle-wasting conditions are also useful. One of the side-effect of being on large doses of steroids, and for long periods of time, is that the sufferer does put on weight. High doses taken for a long time or repeated in short courses can lead to side-effects such as increased risk of infection, thinning of the skin (causing stretch marks), various eye problems such as cataracts or glaucoma, bone thinning or damage, stomach ulcers, irregular monthly periods or, rarely, mental upsets. In children high doses of steroids taken over a long time can stunt growth. But such large doses are reserved for life-threatening conditions when the alternatives are unthinkable.

A wide variety of diseases may need steroid therapy. Some of the main ones are bronchial asthma, rheumatoid arthritis, ulcerative colitis, Crohn's disease, psoriasis and to dampen the potential rejection after organ transplantation.

In order to control the worst symptoms of, say, rheumatoid arthritis (pain, deformity and stiffness) and when all other treatments have failed, steroids or other slow-acting medicines will be required. Steroids tend to be used in the minimum dose which produces the desired effect. If you have to take steroids for a long time your doctor will prescribe as small a dose as possible. Fortunately, many sufferers will have their symptoms controlled sufficiently so that their dose of steroids can be reduced to a low maintenance level that won't increase their weight.

Topical steroids means they are put on the skin. They can reduce the redness and itchiness of certain skin problems and shouldn't be confused with anabolic steroids. They tend to be used for those inflammatory conditions not due to infection, such as eczema. Topical steroids should not be used on large areas of the body for a long time – say, daily for many weeks. Overuse of topical steroids, particularly the stronger ones, may make the skin so thin it can be easily damaged or allow the active ingredient to pass through the skin and affect other parts of the body (especially on the face in infants and children, women who are pregnant, old people and people with kidney problems).

You may be asked to carry a steroid card and if you are, be sure to keep it with you always. You will then be able to show it to any doctor, dentist, nurse or midwife or anyone else who is giving you treatment. Even after your treatment has finished you should tell anyone giving you further treatment that you've had steroid treatment. Your defences may be slow to react as a result. A steroid card may be obtained from your doctor, pharmacist or Local Family Health Service Authority. In Scotland, they are available from the Scottish Office of Home and Health. These enable the correct dose to be continued if you are involved in an accident and taken to hospital unconscious. It can be dangerous to stop high doses of steroids suddenly and, when in shock, the dose may need to be increased since the body needs more at these times.

THRUSH

So many women suffer from thrush without knowing there are a variety of ways to prevent and treat it. Thrush is a common vaginal infection due to the multiplication of a yeast-like fungus known as *candida albicans,* which occurs naturally in the vagina, mouth and digestive tract. When the body's natural balance is upset, perhaps by pregnancy, diabetes, having taken antibiotics recently, having had sex with someone who has thrush or even having a period, the fungus can multiply and cause great irritation and discomfort.

The most common symptoms are soreness, itching and occasionally swelling of the vagina and vulva. There is also often a whitish, curd-like discharge which looks a bit like cottage cheese and has no smell. Sometimes there is a burning feeling at the entrance to the vagina. Sometimes, too, your partner may carry the organism on his penis and develop an itchy rash. If he does, he too should be treated.

There are a number of misconceptions about thrush. It hasn't been scientifically proved that the contraceptive pill causes thrush. It is quite likely that women who are on the pill are getting recurrent attacks because their partners are not using a barrier method of contraception, such as the sheath. This means that the man could be harbouring the thrush under his foreskin and every time they make love he reinfects his partner. This is why it is important for the male partner to be treated at the same time as the woman. All he has to do is rub the cream under the foreskin and around the tip of the penis.

But thrush isn't a venereal disease. It can be sexually transmitted, but virgins have been known to get it. This is because the fungus produces lighter-than-air spores which, should they happen to land on a warm, moist place on the body at the time the person's defences are low, will develop into thrush.

Thrush can be very depressing for the sufferer, but if the rules are followed it can be treated. Many women do suffer numerous attacks of thrush, and once it has been diagnosed by a doctor it can be recognised by the sufferer. But if you experience thrush for the first time, or if you are in any doubt about the condition, always seek the advice of your doctor.

Two new, safe and effective over-the-counter medicines for the treatment of vaginal thrush are now available from pharmacies only. Both Femeron and Canesten 10% VC treat the symptoms of thrush with a convenient, single-dose application. Femeron contains miconazole and Canesten 10% VC contains clotrimazole, which are anti-fungal drugs and should relieve symptoms within two to three days of treatment.

Your doctor may prescribe another form of antifungal cream or pessaries or capsules containing itraconazole (an antifungal agent), taken by mouth. Such preparations continue to work after the capsules have been taken. It may take between a week and a month to reach maximum effect since the medicine remains, working, within these tissues throughout this time, after the capsules have been taken. For thrush, two capsules taken about 12 hours apart from another two, and taken after meals, is therefore the recommended dose that your doctor may prescribe.

Some women find they have recurring attacks, even after being prescribed creams. The reason is that *candida albicans* (thrush) often infects the lower bowel, so even if the vaginal or oral thrush is treated it can recur. There is now a one-day only capsule, Diflucan, which, taken by mouth, is water soluble and therefore gets right into the bloodstream, and is able to destroy the yeast causing the reinfection anywhere in the body. Anti-fungal creams can cause irritation and burning.

There are some very simple things that a woman should and shouldn't do to guard against further attacks of thrush. Make sure you wash every day. When you go to the loo, it's particularly important that you wipe yourself from front to back (not from back to front) after a bowel movement, just as you would do to avoid cystitis. Avoid perfumed soaps, deodorants, bubble baths, etc, which could cause irritation.

Some women have told me that they believe tampons irritate the vagina because of the chemicals in them. Tampons don't contain irritant chemicals. Instead, I believe it is the mere physical presence of the tampons that causes the increased irritation.

Vaginal douches should not be used, although some women do seem to find relief when they insert fresh, live yoghurt into the vagina. This contains 'healthy' germs – the *lactobacilli* which compete with and may overcome the thrush-causing micro-organisms. I'm a great believer in this simple and natural remedy.

Some women have found that using tampons or an intrauterine contraceptive device has put them more at risk of developing thrush. Others have found that wearing synthetic underwear or tight-fitting trousers helps the fungi to thrive because of the warm, moist environment.

If you think you have thrush, you should consult your doctor if any of the following conditions apply: if you haven't had thrush before; if you have a previous history of sexually transmitted disease or exposure to a partner with STD; if you have had more than two previous attacks in the last six months; if you have a known hypersensitivity to Canesten or Femeron; if you are pregnant or think you may be; if you are under 16 or over 60; if you experience any abnormal or irregular vaginal bleeding or blood-stained vaginal discharge, any vaginal sores, ulcers or blisters, any associated lower abdominal pain or difficulty in passing urine; if there is no improvement after seven days of an over-the-counter treatment; if there are any adverse effects such as redness, irritation or swelling associated with any such treatments.

Preparations prescribed Betadine, Canesten, Gyno-Daktarin, Diflucan, Masnoderm, Nizoral, Nystan, Sporanox, Travogyn

TRANQUILLISERS

Both minor and major tranquillisers – those drugs which have been in use for around 30 years or so – have revolutionised the treatment of everyday anxiety and depression as well as the treatment of severe mental illness.

Unfortunately, it's taken us 20 of those 30 years to realise that you don't get measurable benefits from a medicine without getting side-effects and complications. Fortunately, we now know that minor tranquillisers like diazepam (Valium), temazepam (Normison), chlordiazepoxide (Librium) and lorazepam (Ativan) must only be used for the more acute of the everyday anxiety symptoms, for only two weeks or so, and when nothing else will do. If these drugs are used properly and carefully they are of value in these situations.

When anxiety occurs, it will usually be due to either a long-term or recent upset in life. This could be an unhappy relationship, home life, school or work life. When there is a problem that provokes the symptoms it's so much better to deal with that problem whenever it is possible.

Another point is that the major tranquillisers used for long-term mental illness, like schizophrenia, are not to be confused with the minor tranquillisers. The tranquillisers that are used for serious mental illness are vital. Without their use there would be tens of thousands of sufferers who would have to remain in hospital rather than being able to continue enjoying – as many now do – their everyday lives.

So the message is clear. None of us should look to prescribable medicines as a prop for our day-to-day difficulties. Yoga, meditation or relaxation are more natural ways of quelling anxiety when our relationship or work problems, or whatever is causing that anxiety, can't be put right.

THYROID – OVERACTIVE/UNDERACTIVE

When thyroid trouble is firmly diagnosed, doctors will always want to reduce the overactivity by medicines before either operating on the thyroid or treating with a radioactive iodine drink.

A straightforward overactive thyroid gland (hyperthyroidism) is thought to become overactive due to overstimulation by the pituitary gland at the base of the brain. The high activity causes toxic reactions in the body.

The first sign of anything being wrong at all may be a

friend or relative, usually one who hasn't seen the sufferer for some time, commenting upon the 'staring' appearance of their eyes. The following consultation with their doctor will quickly confirm the diagnosis. Such a person may not have suffered the usual symptoms – loss of weight, marked palpitations as the heart overworks, loss of concentration and agitation, shaking hands, and a sudden and increasing tendency to drop things.

Once in a rare while, the thyroid gland will overwork the body to the extent where the heart will fail to work efficiently. The sufferer will then feel acutely breathless and may notice this especially when lying flat in bed at night.

For anyone suffering the sort of symptoms mentioned, it's important to distinguish between an overactive thyroid and the symptoms of everyday anxiety. Many are identical. If you feel that thyroid trouble might be causing your symptoms, then you must see your doctor. A simple blood test will show whether or not you have too high a level of thyroxins. Also, if you do, the thyroid gland may enlarge. It is usually unnoticeable so any enlargement should be investigated by a doctor.

Special anti-thyroid drugs may be used to block the action of the thyroid hormone. An example is carbimazole (Neo Mercazole). Adverse reactions usually occur in the first eight weeks of treatment. The most common minor reactions are nausea, headache, arthralgia, mild gastric distress, skin rashes and pruritis. Hair loss has been occasionally reported. Bone marrow depression has been reported. This means that certain kinds, or all, of the blood's cells – those circulating in the blood – may not be produced in large enough amounts since they're made in the bone marrow.

Drugs to slow the heartbeat are also often needed for a limited time. Such medicines are called beta-blockers, propranolol, for instance (Beta Prograne). Sometimes overactivity doesn't last long and does not recur. In other patients, the overactive thyroid seems to be less controllable and for them, and also in young patients, an operation to remove part of the gland will be advised.

An underactive thyroid (hypothyroidism) seems to happen more often to women than men, usually after the age of 45. It develops slowly as a result of a deficiency of thyroid hormones leading to lack of energy, a thickening and yellow tingeing of the skin, increasing weight, dry lifeless hair and a deeper, croaking voice. Treatment is usually the topping up of the body's thyroid hormone by prescribing thyroxine (Eltroxin). Side-effects may occur when you first start taking this medicine but will reduce as the dosage is lowered to suit your needs. They can include angina pain, irregular heartbeat, diarrhoea, restlessness, excessive loss of weight and muscular weakness.

Preparations prescribed Beta Prograne, Eltroxin, Neo Mercazole

TRAVEL SICKNESS

Symptoms such as nausea and vomiting, loss of appetite, sweating, feeling faint and looking pale, even greenish, during a car, sea or air journey are actually brought on by disturbance to the balance mechanism of the inner ear caused by motion. The movement of the vehicle upsets the link between what the eyes see and what the balance mechanism of the inner ear feels – hence the alternative name of 'motion sickness'. The eyes adjust to the changes in the movement, whereas the inner ear doesn't, so the signals from the eyes and the ears don't quite add up. Medicines for combating travel sickness (motion sickness) are known as anti-emetics. They reduce the sensitivity of the vomiting centre in the brain (see also NAUSEA AND VOMITING, page 115). Patches containing hyoscine (Scopoderm TTS) may be prescribed. These patches are placed on a dry, hairless area of skin behind the ear and need to be worn five to six hours before a journey.

They're designed to last up to three days. When the journey is over you can take off the patch and throw it away. Side-effects of such a medicine can include a dry mouth, sleepiness, dizziness, confusion and hallucination, blurred vision and redness of the skin where a patch has been.

Antihistamines are also used, such as dimenhydrinate (Dramamine) or cinnarizine (Stugeron). They can cause drowsiness, gastrointestinal upsets, allergy and blood disorders.

Preparations prescribed Dramamine, Scopoderm TTS, Stugeron

ULCERS, DUODENAL, GASTRIC AND PEPTIC

There are three types of ulcers discussed in stomach problems – duodenal, gastric and peptic. The last – peptic – is the general name for the common type of ulcer. A gastric ulcer is a peptic ulcer in the stomach and a duodenal ulcer is a peptic ulcer in the duodenum.

Drugs used to treat ulcers are called antacids (see INDIGESTION, page 96) and H2 antagonists which have revolutionised ulcer treatment, and include those such as Tagamet and Galenamet (containing cimetidine) which reduces the secretion of gastric acids and pepsin, that is, the amount of acid in your stomach. Acid plays a part in ulcer disease of the stomach or duodenum so this usually relieves symptoms rapidly and allows the ulcer to heal. Another is Zantac which contains ranitidine and also cuts down the amount of acid in your stomach. Most people taking this type of medicine find they have no problems. For example, more than 35 million patients have been treated with Tagamet world-wide and adverse reactions have been infrequent. Diarrhoea, dizziness or rash, usually mild and short-lived, and tiredness have been reported. Side-effects (uncommon) of Zantac include headache, dizziness, skin, jaundice or confusion. Other H2 antagonists are famotidine (Pepcid) and nizatidine (Axid).

Sometimes ulcers can be caused as a consequence of other drug treatments such as arthritis treated by non-steroidal anti-inflammatory drugs. There are two newer medicines prescribed for this particular problem, in addition to H2 antagonists. They are misoprostol (Cytotec) or omeprazole (Losec). Cytotec is an analogue (similar chemicially and in function) of naturally occurring prostaglandin E1 which promotes peptic ulcer healing and symptomatic relief. Diarrhoea has been reported and is occasionally severe and prolonged and may need withdrawal of the drug. Losec is a specific inhibitor of the gastric proton pump (H, K+ATPase) in the parietal cell. This means that the normal way in which chemicals work with the acid-producing parietal cells in the stomach lining are inhibited. By inhibiting the movements of these chemicals – called the proton pump mechanism – the symptoms and conditions provoked by acid overproduction are successfully controlled.

I'm often asked whether it's possible to have an ulcer without pain and is it more dangerous? Yes, a stomach ulcer can occur without pain. Although some of the more serious ones can be pain-free, they are rarely symptom-free. When an ulcer is painless and potentially dangerous, the sufferer will often have completely lost his or her appetite and, as a result, have also lost quite a bit of weight by the time the ulcer is diagnosed.

Interestingly, research at Manchester Royal Infirmary suggests that people who drink their tea and coffee very hot are more likely to develop peptic ulcers than those who have their drinks cooler. Temperatures above 60°C can adversely alter the protective mucus that lines the gut and many people with gut disorders were found regularly to take their drinks at temperatures between 62°C and 73°C, whereas the healthy group preferred theirs at 56°C. Man is the only creature who chooses to eat and drink at temperatures well above normal body temperature and it appears that this insistence on things being 'piping hot' is not such a good idea after all.

Preparations prescribed Aluhyde, Antepsin, Axid, Biogastrone, Cytotec, De-Nol Tablets/Liquid, De-Noltab, Diovol, Dyspamet, Galenamet, Gastrobid Continus, Gastrozepin, Kolanticon Gel, Losec, Maalox TC Suspension and Tablets, Mucogel, Pepcid, Tagamet, Zantac

URTICARIA

More often known as hives or nettle rash, urticaria is a very common skin condition which affects one in five people at some time in their lives. Women are particularly prone, perhaps because of hormonal influences. With 'ordinary' urticaria, weals – intensely itchy raised marks on the surface of the skin – suddenly develop. They are usually short-lived, lasting for a few hours or days, but may last longer. The weals can be any size, appear anywhere on the sufferer's body and may be numerous. They are usually pale in the middle and red around the edges and are due to dilation of the capillaries – small blood vessels under the skin – which makes their walls more permeable and enables clear fluid called serum to leak out. If enough serum leaks out, blisters may form.

If deeper tissues are involved, a more severe type of urticaria known as angio-oedema may occur. Then the swellings are much larger, commonly affecting the face, eyelids, hands, forearms and throat and sometimes causing serious breathing difficulties. Joints in the arms and legs may also become inflamed and painful. About half the people who suffer from ordinary urticaria have recurrent attacks of angio-oedema too.

So what causes this reaction in the blood vessels? Often it is due to an increased circulation of histamine, a chemical normally present in the body. This increase can be triggered by many factors, including various foods, drugs and inhalants such as pollens, house dust and animal 'dander' (skin flakes which the animal sheds naturally and various chemicals which its body gives off). Two foods that are frequently responsible are shellfish and strawberries – so urticaria is a hazard of summer for those susceptible. Other foods that may produce the reaction include eggs, nuts, chocolate, tomatoes, pork, milk and yeast. Artificial colourings and preservatives can do so, too.

Aspirin can also be a cause of urticaria, or it can aggravate it. Penicillin is another possible culprit, as are the non-steroidal anti-inflammatory drugs often given to treat arthritis. Sometimes contact with certain substances will bring the symptoms on – cosmetics are one example. Insect stings can also cause this type of reaction, which may even be life-threatening if the breathing is affected (see BITES AND STINGS, page 32).

People whose urticaria occurs in response to triggers such as these are often but not always allergy-prone individuals – sufferers from hay fever, asthma or eczema for example – and the tendency can run in families. Anxiety may also play a part.

Other constituents in the body – called catecholamines – can, by irritating the tissues surrounding them, have the same effect on the blood vessels as histamine, and almost anything can act as the trigger in this allergic-type of urticaria. I had it once after eating raw fish in a foreign restaurant, for example, but it may also have been due to the monosodium glutamate used as a taste-enhancer.

It can therefore be exceedingly difficult to track down the cause, in order to avoid it if the attacks are recurrent. In fact three out of four people are unable to do so, in spite of persistent detective work.

Some more unusual forms of urticaria have a physical cause. Cold winds or rain, or just immersing the hands or bathing in cold water, can cause weals to appear in susceptible people. If an ice cube on the skin produces a weal, this confirms the diagnosis of 'cold urticaria' – the type that's induced by the cold.

Some people develop weals when exposed to sunlight – 'solar urticaria' – or deep, painful, non-itchy swellings which occur about two hours after some particular pressure on the skin. The hands may swell, for instance, after carrying a heavy shopping bag, or the balls of the feet after spending some time on a ladder.

Another strange form of urticaria is called dermographism, loosely 'translated' as skin writing. A mild, stroking pressure – with a fingernail for example – will produce a temporary, raised line with reddened edges. The skin can literally be used as a drawing board.

Fortunately, however, most cases of urticaria tend to resolve themselves in due course, and in the meantime antihistamine tablets prescribed by your doctor usually relieve the symptoms (see also HAY FEVER, page 81). If angio-oedema is severe and breathing becomes difficult, emergency treatment by injection may be necessary to reduce the swelling.

Urticaria can occur as part of some other underlying condition – thyroid disease, for example. So if the cause is not immediately apparent, or you have more than one attack, or are concerned, do consult your doctor. He or she may wish to do blood tests and other investigations or refer you to a skin specialist.

Preparations prescribed Dimotane LA/Tablets/Elixir, Piriton Tablets, Piriton Injection, Primalan, Tavegil, Vallergan

VERTIGO AND MENIÈRE'S DISEASE

Menière's Disease or Syndrome is a very distressing condition affecting the hearing and balance of about 25,000 people in Britain. It usually develops between the ages of 30 and 60, affects men and women equally and one in 20 of those will have a fellow-sufferer in the family.

Deep inside the ear, a system of intercommunicating, fluid-filled channels and cavities – called the labyrinth – normally controls our balance and hearing. The symptoms of Menière's Disease, which include vertigo (giddiness), vomiting, tinnitus (ringing in the ears) and loss of hearing, are due to a disturbance in the fluid-regulating mechanism within the labyrinth. The amount of fluid there increases, leading to distention, a feeling of fullness and the other symptoms already described. What causes the disturbance however is still uncertain.

Many specialists believe that changes in the blood vessels (similar to those that occur during a migraine) are responsible, with fluctuation in blood supply to the inner ear – a theory backed by the fact that one in three of those with Menières are also migraine sufferers. Other suggested causes include a blockage in the usual drainage system in the labyrinth, altered fluid absorption there, an allergy, or a fault in the body's immune system (called an auto-immune reaction) whereby antibodies in the blood which normally protect us against disease attack, in this case, the delicate tissues of the inner ear.

The first symptoms of Menières disease may pass almost unnoticed and be soon forgotten – perhaps just a slight tinnitus and feeling of fullness in one ear (it is unusual for both ears to be affected) lasting a day or two. It may be weeks, months or even years before any further symptoms occur. Vertigo develops in later attacks, often coming on suddenly, and sometimes waking the person from sleep. Even when lying still, they may feel as if their whole body is moving about or as if everything is moving around them. Nausea and vomiting can also be very distressing. The amount of hearing loss will vary from person to person and although it frequently improves as the attack subsides, some deafness usually remains. Attacks can last anything from 15 minutes to 12 hours and often occur in clusters over several days or weeks with long periods of remission in between. They tend to become less frequent and severe in time and may 'burn themselves out' completely.

Many other conditions can cause symptoms similar to Menière's disease and in order to exclude them quite prolonged specialist investigations may be necessary. If the ear is examined between attacks, nothing abnormal may be found. When Menière's is diagnosed, most sufferers find that medicines prescribed by the doctor control their symptoms and a combination of different tablets may be used. Some dilate the blood vessels, some increase the output of urine (both, indirectly, diminish the excess fluid in the ear and so the giddiness and deafness) and others relieve the vomiting.

Cutting down on salt in your diet may also help. If hearing is badly affected or threatened, or the vertigo does not respond to medicines, there are various techniques a surgeon can suggest.

Preparations prescribed Dramamine, Serc, Serc-16, Stemetil, Stemetil Eff, Valoid

WORMS

I regularly receive letters from people who are puzzled when they experience intense itching, just around the anus, and nothing that they do – whether showering or using cream – seems to get rid of it. Sometimes the discomfort makes life almost impossible. Yet they are so embarrassed about it they can't bring themselves to discuss the problem with their doctor.

If this happens to you, you should really go to your doctor to discover the cause of your itching if it persists for any length of time. It's highly likely, though, that you have threadworms. They're a very common problem and do tend to cause an itchy bottom, especially first thing in the morning.

Threadworms (*enterobius*) are like wriggling threads of white cotton – hence the name. They are less than 1.5 cm long and can be seen wriggling in the faeces. Horrible as they sound, they are a very common problem, particularly in children. It is estimated that up to 40% of children below the age of ten are infected with threadworms, though many may not show the 'itching' symptoms generally associated with them.

Threadworms produce large numbers of tiny eggs that cannot readily be seen with the naked eye. The eggs are present in house dust, they stick to clothing, carpets, towels and bed linen and can also be picked up, in heavily infected households, from food on which eggs have been 'hand deposited' or settled. They are also spread by hand contact. If another person should touch an infected person's hands when eggs are present and subsequently put his or her hands into the mouth, then he or she will also become infected as a result of swallowing the eggs. The eggs then hatch in the lower bowel and at night a female worm starts to lay her eggs just outside the anus. She can lay up to 10,000 eggs, which can cause severe itching.

The wriggling of threadworms irritates the anus and their presence slightly inflames it. This normally makes the sufferer scratch and so pick up eggs on the hands and under the fingernails. The most common sign of threadworms is scratching of the bottom, particularly at night and first thing in the morning. When the scratching takes place solely during the night, as sometimes happens, it may just cause a disturbance of sleep and hence daytime irritability – the itching itself may not be apparent. Some sufferers show no signs of infection, in which case it is a question of spotting the worms in the motions in order to detect their presence.

You can use a mirror to check whether you can see any worms on yourself. Remember they look like fine, moving white threads. Of course, even if you can't see them immediately, it's still possible that you have them.

Threadworms are very common and appear even in the cleanest households, so there's no need to feel embarrassed about consulting your doctor. They only affect humans, never pets. And although they can be uncomfortable, they are generally harmless and do not usually cause any long-term damage.

Medicines contain mebendazole (Vermox), thiabendazole (Mintezol) or piperazine (Pripsen). These treatments are usually effective, but you should follow the instructions on the packet exactly. If the problem recurs, then everyone in your household should take a course of the medicine at the same time, as they may be harbouring worms themselves without necessarily having any symptoms. If this is that case, the worms can, in a variety of ways, be continually passed from person to person. So if, after treatment, your symptoms return, gather your courage and bring up the subject with everyone sharing your home – you may find they've been suffering silently, too.

Make sure that everyone scrubs their fingers and nails with a brush after each visit to the toilet and before each meal. Disinfect – by washing thoroughly – the toilet seat, toilet handle or chain and door handle regularly, as well as making sure you dust and vacuum bedrooms thoroughly.

Roundworms (ascariasis) can also be treated by piperazine. These worms are one of the largest parasites. They can be 10–30 cm long, look like earthworms and can block the intestine. They're transmitted by eggs found in contaminated raw food or in soil. Fortunately, they're rare. The sufferer may inexplicably lose weight or suffer other symptoms – a cough is not uncommon. When the doctor takes a blood test, the results should strongly suggest the diagnosis. Occasionally, an adult worm, not unlike an earthworm, may be passed in the faeces or even vomited up. But don't be alarmed – as I said, it's rare, thank goodness.

The roundworm is usually eradicated by a single dose of a medicine containing piperazine, whereas threadworms may need several days' treatment, as instructed, and phases of treatment may sometimes be separated by a week or more.

Preparations prescribed Mintezol, Pripsen, Vermox

A–Z of Medicines

Accupro
Tablets containing quinapril (an ACE inhibitor) for the treatment of high blood pressure. PARKE DAVIS

Accuretic
Tablets containing quinapril (an ACE inhibitor) and hydrochlorothiazide for the treatment of high blood pressure. PARKE DAVIS

Actinac
Lotion containing chloramphenicol, hydrocortisone acetate, butoxyethyl nicotinate, allantoin and precipitated sulphur for the treatment of acne. ROUSSEL

Adcortyl in Orabase
Paste containing triamcinolone acetonide. Uses include aphthous ulcers. SQUIBB

Adizem
Tablets containing dilitiazem hydrochloride (a calcium antagonist) for high blood pressure and angina. NAPP

AeroBec
Inhalation therapy providing beclomethasone dipropionate for asthma and bronchitis. 3M HEALTH CARE

Aerocrom Inhaler
An inhaler designed for patients who have been shown to need regular doses of sodium cromoglycate and salbutamol for the treatment of their asthma. FISONS

Aerolin
Inhalation therapy providing salbutamol for asthma and bronchitis. 3M HEALTH CARE

Alcoderm Cream/Lotion
A liquid paraffin lotion for dry, chafed or irritated skin.

Alcoderm can be used in any condition where the moisture content of the horny layer has decreased below the normal level and the skin is no longer soft and pliable. GALDERMA (UK) LTD

Aldactide 50/25
Tablets containing spironolactone and hydroflumethiazide. Aldactide is a potassium-conserving diuretic with antihypertensive activity. It's recommended for the treatment of high blood pressure and for the control of oedema in congestive cardiac failure. GOLD CROSS

Algesal
Cream containing diethylamine salicylate (an analgesic) for the symptomatic relief of rheumatic and minor musculo-skeletal conditions including lumbago, fibrositis, sciatica, bruises and sprains. DUPHAR

Algicon Tablets and Suspension
Tablets or suspension containing magnesium alginate, aluminium hydroxide/magnesium carbonate co-gel, magnesium carbonate and potassium bicarbonate for the relief of heartburn associated with gastric reflux, reflux oesophagitis, hiatus hernia, pregnancy and hyperacidity. RHONE-POULENC RORER

Alomide
Opthalmic solution containing lodoxamide used to treat non-infectious conjunctivitis probably caused by an allergy. GALEN LTD

Aloxiprin
A non-narcotic analgesic that is a form of aspirin.

Alphaderm Cream
Cream containing hydrocortisone for the treatment of dry eczematous skin conditions. PROCTER & GAMBLE

Alphodith
A range of ointments containing dithranol for the treatment of psoriasis including of the scalp. STAFFORD-MILLER

Alphosyl
Lotion and cream containing coal tar and allantoin for the treatment of psoriasis and psoriasis of the scalp. STAFFORD-MILLER

Alphosyl HC Cream
Cream containing coal tar, allantoin and hydrocortisone for the treatment of psoriasis. STAFFORD-MILLER

Alu-Cap
Aluminium hydroxide gel an antacid. 3M HEALTH CARE

Aluhyde
Antacid and antispasmodic tablets containing dried aluminium hydroxide gel, magnesium trisilicate and belladonna liq. for the relief of functional dyspepsia, gastritis, reflux oesophagitis and gastric and duodenal ulcer. SINCLAIR PHARMACEUTICALS

Alupent
Tablets, syrup, metered aerosol containing orciprenaline sulphate (a medicine which acts like the body's own 'automatic' nervous system chemicals). It dilates the bronchial tubes for the relief of bronchospasm, as in asthma, bronchitis and emphysema. BOEHRINGER INGELHEIM

Alvedon Suppositories
Suppositories containing paracetamol for the treatment of mild to moderate pain and a raised temperature in children.
ASTRA PHARMACEUTICALS LTD

Alvercol
Granules containing sterculia (a water absorbing vegetable gum) and alverine citrate (an antispasmodic agent) for the treatment of muscle spasm disorders of the colon and irritable bowel syndrome.
NORGINE

Ambaxin
Tablets containing bacampicillin hydrochloride (an antibacterial) uses include sinusitis, tonsilitis, bronchitis, skin and soft tissue infections, otitis media. UPJOHN LTD

ammonium chloride
An expectorant used for coughs.

Amoxil
Capsules, tablets, syrups, sachets, paediatric suspension and vials for injection containing amoxycillin – a broad spectrum antibiotic for the treatment of commonly occurring bacterial infections.
BENCARD

Amoxycillin
A broad spectrum antibiotic for the treatment of commonly occurring bacterial infections available as a generic.

Amfipen Capsules/Syrup/Syrup Forte
Capsules or syrup containing ampicillin (an antibiotic) for a wide range of infections such as ear, nose and throat infections; bronchitis; pneumonia; urinary tract

infections, gastro-intestinal infections; enteric fevers such as typhoid fever and in the treatment of gonorrhoea. BROCADES

Amytal
Tablets containing amylobarbitone for the treatment of severe, intractable insomnia. LILLY

Anacal
Suppositories or ointment containing mucopoly-saccharide (a complex carbohydrate), polysulphuric acid ester (Heparinoid) and oxypolyethoxydodecane (Lauromacrogol 400) for the relief of symptoms associated with piles, anal itching and inflammation. PANPHARMA

Anafranil/Anafranil SR
Tablets, capsules, syrup, ampoules of clomipramine hydrochloride (an antidepressant) for symptoms of depressive illness especially where sedation is needed. GEIGY

Antepsin
Tablets and suspension containing sucralfate. Uses include the treatment of ulcers and chronic gastritis. WYETH

Anthranol
Ointments of differing strength containing dithranol for psoriasis including psoriasis of the scalp. STIEFEL

Anturan
Tablets containing sulphinpyrazone to treat gout. GEIGY

Anugesic – HC Cream and Suppositories
Soothing, antiseptic, steroid product containing pramoxine hydrochloride, hydrocortisone acetate, benzyl benzoate, bismuth oxide, balsam peru, and zinc oxide for piles. PARKE-DAVIS

Anusol
Cream containing bismuth oxide, balsam peru and zinc oxide for the treatment of piles. Ointment and suppositories also contain bismuth subgallate. PARKE-DAVIS

Apresoline
Tablets containing hydralazine hydrochloride (a vasodilator) used to treat high blood pressure. CIBA

Aquadrate Cream
Cream containing urea for the management of chronic dry skin conditions. PROCTER & GAMBLE

Arelix Capsules
Capsules containing piretanide, a diuretic for the treatment of high blood pressure. HOECHST

Arthitrex
Tablets containing methotrexate for rheumatoid arthritis. LEDERLE

Arthrotec
Tablets containing diclofenac sodium (a non-steroidal anti-inflammatory drug) and misoprostol (a gastroduodenal mucosal protective agent) for the treatment of rheumatoid arthritis and osteoarthritis where prevention of drug-induced gastric and duodenal ulceration is needed. GOLD CROSS

Arthroxen
Tablets containing naproxen for the treatment of arthritis, gout and acute musculoskeletal disorders.
CP PHARMACEUTICALS

Asacol
Tablets and suppositories containing mesalazine for the treatment of ulcerative colitis.
SMITH KLINE AND FRENCH

Ascabiol
An emulsion containing benzyl benzoate (an acaricide) used in the treatment of scabies. Also used for pediculosis (lice infestation).
RHONE-POULENC RORER

Asendis
Tablets containing amoxapine, an antidepressant for the symptomatic treatment of depression. CYANIMID

Aspirin
A non-narcotic analgesic which has anti-inflammatory properties to relieve mild to moderate pain and reduce fever.

Ativan Tablets (Generic on the NHS)
Tablets containing lorazepam (a benzodiazepine) for the short-term treatment of anxiety. Can also be used as premedication before operative dentistry and as a sedative for the anxious dental patient, and as premedication before general surgery. WYETH

Atromid
Capsules containing clofibrate for high cholesterol.
ICI

Atrovent, Atrovent Forte Metered Dose Inhaler, Nebuliser Solution
Metered dose inhalers and solution containing ipraropium bromide (a

bronchodilator), for the treatment of chronic reversible airways obstruction, particularly in chronic bronchitis. BOEHRINGER INGELHEIM

Avloclor Tablets
An antimalarial drug containing chloroquine phosphate used in the treatment of rheumatoid arthritis, as well as malaria, lupus and treatment of amoebic hepatitis and abscess. ICI

Avomine
Tablets containing promethazine theoclate (an anti-emetic) for the prevention and treatment of nausea and vomiting as a result of various causes including travel sickness, vertigo due to Menière's syndrome and labyrinthitis.
RHONE-POULENC RORER

Audax
Ear drops containing Mundicylat brand of choline salicylate for relief of ear pain in acute and chronic *otitis media* and *externa*. NAPP

Augmentin
Tablets and suspension containing the antibioitic co-amoxiclav (amoxycillin with clavulanic acid), a broad spectrum antibiotic for the treatment of commonly occurring bacterial infections. It can also be administered intravenously. BEECHAM RESEARCH

Bactrim
Drapsules (capsuliform, film-coated tablets), tablets, dispersible tablets, suspension and paediatric syrup containing trimethoprim and sulphamethoxazole. Uses include respiratory tract infections, genito-urinary tract infections, gastro-intestinal infections. ROCHE

Bactroban Nasal
An ointment containing calcium mupirocin, a topical antibacterial agent used to treat infections in and around the nostrils. BEECHAM RESEARCH

Bactroban Ointment
Ointment containing mupirocin a topical antibacterial agent, active against those organisms responsible for the majority of skin infections, for example impetigo, folliculitis, furunculosis. BEECHAM RESEARCH

Balneum
A liquid containing soya oil (an emollient) for the treatment of dry skin conditions including dermatitis and eczema. MERCK

Balneum Plus
A bath oil containing soya oil and mixed lauromacrogols which means it has emollient and local anaesthetic properties and provides relief of pruritis (itching). It's recommended for the treatment of dry skin conditions including those associated with dermatitis and eczema where pruritis is also experienced. MERCK

Balneum with Tar
Bath oil with soya oil and coal tar distillate for the treatment of eczema, psoriasis, dandruff, pruritic dermatoses and ichthysosis – severe dryness of the skin. MERCK

Baltar Shampoo
A shampoo containing coar tar distillate for the treatment of scalp disorders such as psoriarsis, eczema, dandruff, seborrhoeic and pruritic dermatoses. MERCK

Becloforte
Inhaler and diskhaler providing beclomethasone dipropionate for the treatment of asthma.
ALLEN & HANBURYS

Beconase
Aqueous nasal spray and nasal spray containing beclomethasone dipropionate for the prevention and treatment of perennial and seasonal allergic rhinitis.
ALLEN & HANBURYS

Becotide
Inhaler, rotacaps and suspension for nebulisation containing beclomethasone dipropionate for the treatment of asthma.
ALLEN & HANBURYS

Bellocarb (Not on the NHS)
Prolonged acting antacid tablets with mild purgative effect due to the presence of magnesium, containing belladonna extract, magnesium trisilicate, and magnesium carbonate. Used in the management of gastric and duodenal ulcers where intermittent constipation has been a problem. SINCLAIR

Benemid
Tablets containing probenecid for the treatment of gout. MERCK SHARP & DOHME LTD

Benoral
Suspension, granules or tablets containing benorylate, an anti-inflammatory analgesic and antipyretic for the treatment of arthritis and painful musculo-skeletal conditions. SANOFI WINTHROP

Benorylate
An anti-inflammatory analgesic used to treat arthritis and painful musculo-skeletal conditions.

Benzagel 5 & 10
Gel containning benzoyl peroxide for the treatment of acne. BIOGLAN

benzoin tincture
Add to boiling water as an inhalation for the common cold.

Berotec 100/200
Metered dose inhalers containing fenoterol hydrobromide for reversible airways obstruction as in bronchial asthma, bronchitis and emphysema.
BOEHRINGER INGELHEIM

Berotec Nebuliser Solution
Solution containing sodium metabisulphite and disodium edetate uses as Berotec.
BOEHRINGER INGELHEIM

Betaloc
Tablets containing metoprolol tartrate (a beta-blocker). Uses include the management of high blood pressure, angina, abnormal heart rhythms and the prevention of migraine.
ASTRA

Betaloc SA
Tablets containing metoprolol tartrate (a beta-blocker) for the management of angina and high blood pressure and for the prevention of migraine. ASTRA

Beta Prograne
Capsules containing propranolol hydrochloride (a beta-blocker) for the control of high blood pressure, the management of angina, anxiety and essential tremor and for the prevention of migraine, and for the management of thyrotoxicosis – an over-active thyroid gland. Also available as Half Beta-Prograne.
TILLOMED LABORATORIES LTD

Betnovate Cream/Lotion/ Ointment
Strong and rapidly effective treatments containing betamethasone (a topical steroid) for inflamed skin conditions such as eczema, dermatitis and psoriasis.
GLAXO

Betnovate-N Ointment
Ointment containing betamethasone (a topical steroid) and antibacterial agent neomycin sulphate. A strong and rapidly effective treatment for inflamed skin

conditions such as eczema, dermatitis and psoriasis in which infection may be a problem. GLAXO

Betnovate RD Ointment
Ointment containing betamethasone (a topical steroid) which contains less active ingredient than Betnovate Ointment for inflamed skin conditions such as eczema, dermatitis and psoriasis. GLAXO

Betnovate Rectal Ointment
Ointment containing betamethasone valerate (a topical steroid), lignocaine hydrochloride (a local anaesthetic), and phenylephrine hydrochloride (a vasoconstrictor) – a strong preparation for the rapid relief of discomfort, pain, itchiness or irritation around the back passage due to piles. GLAXO

Binovum
Oral contraceptive containing norethisterone and ethinyloestradiol. ORTHO

Biogastrone
Tablets containing carbenoxolone sodium for the treatment of benign gastric ulcers in young and middle-aged patients, i.e. those wiin the age range of 16 to 65 years. SANOFI WINTHROP

Bioplex
Mouthwash containing carbenoxolone sodium for the treatment of mouth ulcers. THAMES LABORATORIES

Biorphen
Solution containing orphenadrine hydrochloride, an anticholinergic preparation for the treatment of Parkinson's disease. BIOGLAN

bisacodyl
A stimulant laxative used for constipation.

Blocadren
Tablets containing timolol maleate (a beta-blocker) to treat high blood pressure, angina and for prevention of migraine. MERCK SHARP & DOHME LTD

Bonjela Oral Pain-Relieving Gel
Gel containing choline salicylate, a pain-reliever, and cetalkonium chloride, an antiseptic, in a sugar-free base, for the relief of the pain and discomfort of common mouth ulcers, cold sores, denture spots and infant teething. RECKITT & COLMAN

Bradilan
Tablets containing tetranicotinoylfructose for high cholesterol. NAPP

Brevinor
Combined oral contraceptive containing norethisterone and ethinyloestradiol. SYNTEX

Bricanyl Inhaler, Bricanyl Spacer Inhaler (aerosols); Bricanyl Tablets, Syrup; Bricanyl Respules, Respirator Solution (solution for nebulisation); Bricanyl Sa (tablets); Bricanyl Turboinhaler (powder inhaler)
Bricanyl range contains terbutaline sulphate, a bronchodilator recommended for the relief and prevention of bronchospasm in bronchial asthma and in chronic bronchitis, emphysema and other broncho-pulmonary disorders. ASTRA

Brocadopa Capsules
Capsules containing levodopa for the treatment of all forms of Parkinson's disease except drug- induced. BROCADES

Broflex
Syrup containing benzhexol hydrochloride, a parasympatholytic drug – a medicine which provides its beneficial effect by mimicking part of the body's autonomic (automatic) nervous system. It is used in the treatment of Parkinson's disease. BIOGLAN

Brufen
Tablets, granules or syrup containing ibuprofen for the treatment of arthritis, bursitis etc, low back pain, soft-tissue injuries, period pain, dental pain and migraine. BOOTS

Buccastem
Tablets containing prochlorperazine maleate (a powerful phenothiazine neuroleptic, i.e from the group of medicines used to treat severe mental disorders like schizophrenia) for the symptomatic treatment of vertigo due to Menière's disease, labyrinthitis and other causes; for nausea and vomiting from whatever cause and in the treatment of migraine. RECKITT & COLMAN

Buscopan
Tablets containing hyoscine-N-butylbromide (an antispasmodic agent) uses include bowel spasm and period pain. BOEHRINGER INGELHEIM

Buspar
Tablets containing buspirone hydrochloride for the

short-term management of anxiety.

BRISTOL-MYERS PHARMACEUTICALS

Cacit Tablets

Tablets containing calcium carbonate. Uses include slowing down of bone demineralisation in osteoporosis. PROCTER & GAMBLE

Calpol Infant Suspension

Suspension containing paracetamol for the treatment of mild to moderate pain and fever. WELLCOME

Calsynar

Injections of synthetic salmon calcitonin. Uses include osteoporosis. Studies have shown that it may be effective in the prevention of progressive loss of bone mass in the treatment of postmenopausal osteoporosis. RHONE-POULENC RORER

Camcolit

Tablets and controlled release tablets containing lithium carbonate: an anti-depressant.

NORGINE

Canesten/Canesten HC

Cream containing clotrimazole (an antifungal agent) and HC, hydrocortisone (a topical corticosteroid). Uses include the treatment of itchy and inflamed fungal skin infections. BAYER

Capasal

Shampoo containing salicylic acid, coconut oil and distilled coal tar for dry scaly scalp conditions and cradle cap.

DERMAL

Caprin

Intestinal release aspirin tablets (containing acetylsalicylic acid) used as an antipyretic – a temperature-lowering, anti-inflammatory and analgesic agent designed to reduce the gastric side-effects of aspirin in rheumatoid arthritis and in other conditions needing continued management with aspirin. Caprin may also be used to reduce the risk of myocardial infarction in patients with unstable angina or in patients with previous history of myocardial infarction. This is the medical way of saying that a heart attack, a coronary thrombosis, has left a part of the heart's muscle damaged, usually permanently.

SINCLAIR PHARMACEUTICALS

Carbalax

Suppositories containing sodium acid phosphate anhydrous and sodium bicarbonate for constipation and other conditions such as when there is a need to keep stools to normal consistency when a patient is suffering from piles. PHARMAX

Cardinol
Tablets containing propranolol hydrochloride – uses include the control of high blood pressure, angina, and the prevention of migraine. CP PHARMACEUTICALS

Carisoma
Tablets containing carisoprodol, used as a sedative as an adjunct to the symptomatic treatment of acute musculoskeletal disorders with painful muscle spasm. PHARMAX

Carylderm
Lotion or shampoo containing carbaryl for the treatment of head and pubic lice. NAPP

Catapres
Tablets, capsules, ampoules, containing clonidine hydrochloride for high blood pressure, high blood pressure in pregnancy and hypertensive crises. BOEHRINGER INGELHEIM

Celectol Tablets
Tablets containing celiprolol hydrochloride for the management of mild to moderate high blood pressure. RHONE-POULENC RORER

Celevac Tablets
Tablets containing methylcellulose (which absorbs water to swell to a soft gel of uniform consistency). Uses include the management of diverticular disease and constipation. BOEHRINGER INGELHEIM

Ceporex Capsules/ Paediatric Drops/ Suspension/Syrup/ Tablets
Antibiotic treatments containing cephalexin. Uses include the treatment of respiratory tract infections, ear, nose and throat infections, skin and soft tissue infections, gonorrhoea. GLAXO

Cerumol Ear Drops
Ear drops containing paradichlorobenzene, an insecticide, chlorbutol, which has antibacterial properties, and arachis oil – for the loosening and removal of ear wax. LABORATORIES FOR APPLIED BIOLOGY

Cetavlex Cream
A cream containing cetrimide (an antiseptic) for skin disorders such as minor wounds, burns, abrasions and nappy rash. ICI

chlordiazepoxide
A long-acting benzodiaepine used to treat anxiety.

Chloromycetin
Capsules or suspension containing chloramphenicol (an antibiotic) used for serious infections. PARKE DAVIS

Chloromycetin Hydrocortisone Ophthalmic Ointment
Ointment containing chloramphenicol and hydrocortisone acetate for eye inflammation due to allergy when there is also a bacterial infection. PARKE DAVIS

Chloromyctin Ophthalmic Preparations
Eye drops or ointment containing chloramphenicol (an antibiotic) for the treatment of bacterial conjunctivitis. PARKE DAVIS

Choledyl
Tablets containing choline theophyllinate for the relief and prevention of bronchospasm in chronic bronchitis and asthma. PARKE DAVIS

Cicatrin
Broad-spectrum antibacterial aerosol, powder and cream containing neomycin sulphate, zinc bacitracin, I-cysteine and glycine (powder and cream also dl-threonine) for bacterial skin infections. WELLCOME

Cidomycin (Topical)
Wide spectrum antibiotic cream or ointment containing gentamicin sulphate for the treatment of bacterial skin infections and infected dermatitis, pustular acne, infected burns and wounds, ulcers and paronychia – infections under or close to the nails. ROUSSEL

Cidomycin Eye/Ear Drops or Ointment
Antibiotic preparations containing gentamicin sulphate. Uses include bacterial infections of the eye and external ear infections. ROUSSEL

Cilest 250/35
Combined oral contraceptive containing norgestimate and ethinyloestradiol. ORTHO

Clarityn Tablets/Syrup
Tablets and syrup containing loratadine (an antihistamine) for hay fever, perennial allergic rhinitis, and urticaria. SCHERING-PLOUGH

Climagest
Hormone replacement therapy for the treatment of

menopausal symptoms providing both oestrogen and progestogen. SANDOZ

Clinoril/Clinoril 200
Tablets containing sulindac (a nonsteroidal analgesic/anti-inflammatory agent with antipyretic – temperature lowering – properties) for the treatment of osteoarthritis, rheumatoid arthritis, ankylosing spondylitis, acute gouty arthritis and disorders such as bursitis, tendinitis, and tenosynovitis.
MERCK SHARP & DOHME LTD

Clozaril
Tablets containing clozapine used to treat the symptoms of schizophrenia. SANDOZ

Co-Betaloc
Tablets containing metoprolol tartrate (a beta-blocker) for the management of high blood pressure. ASTRA

Co-Betaloc SA
Tablets containing metoprolol tartrate (a beta-blocker) and hydrochlorothiazide (a diuretic) for the manaement of high blood pressure. ASTRA

co-codamol
An analgesic containing the opiate codeine phosphate and paracetamol for the treatment of pain.

co-codaprin
An analgesic containing the opiate codeine phosphate with aspirin for the treament of pain.

Codafen Continus
Tablets containing ibuprofen and codeine phosphate for the relief of pain in arthritis and other inflammatory disorders.
NAPP

co-danthramer/co-danthrusate
A faecal softener/stimulant used for constipation.

codeine phosphate
An opiate, and narcotic analgesic which is also used as a cough suppressant.

codeine linctus
A cough suppressant.

co-dydramol
An analgesic containing dihydrocodeine and paracetamol.

co-proxamol
An analgesic containing paracetamol and dextropropoxyphene.

Cogentin
Tablets containing benztropine mesylate (an anti-parkinsonian agent with powerful anticholinergic

effects) for symptomatic treatment of Parkinson's disease. MERCK SHARP & DOHME LTD

Colestid
Granules and powder containing colestipol hydrochloride for high cholesterol. UPJOHN

Colifoam
Foam containing hydrocortisone acetate – anti-inflammatory corticosteroid therapy for the topical treatment of ulcerative colitis. STAFFORD-MILLER

Concordin
Tablets containing protriptyline hydrochloride for the symptoms of depression. MERCK SHARP & DOHME LTD

Conotrone
Cream containing benzalkonium chloride (an antiseptic) and dimethicone (a water repellent) used for protection of the skin from moisture, irritants, chafing and contamination with bacteria or yeasts, as in the prevention and treatment of nappy rash, pressure sores and in the management of incontinence. BOEHRINGER INGELHEIM

Conova 30
A combined oral contraceptive containing ethynodiol diacetate (a progestogen) and ethinyloestradiol (an oestrogen). GOLD CROSS

Corsodyl Dental Gel/ Mouthwash/Mint Mouthwash/Spray
Gel and mouthwash containing chlorhexidine gluconate as an aid in the treatment and prevention of gingivitis and in the maintenance of oral hygiene. It's also useful in the management of mouth ulcers. ICI

Cremalgin Balm
Balm containing methyl nicotinate, capiscin and glycol salicylate for the symptomatic relief of rheumatism, sciatica, lumbago, fibrositis and muscular stiffness. RHONE-POULENC RORER

Cyclo-Progynova
Hormone replacement therapy containing oestradiol valerate and levonorgestrel. SCHERING

Cyklokapron Tablets
Tablets containing tranexamic acid – uses include the treatment of menorrhagia. KABI PHARMACIA

Cymalon
Granules containing sodium citrate, citric acid, sodium bicarbonate and sodium carbonate for the relief of symptoms of cystitis.

STERLING HEALTH

Cytotec
Tablets containing misoprostol for the healing of duodenal ulcers and gastric ulcers, including those induced by non-steroidal anti-inflammatory drugs in arthritic patients at risk, while continuing their NSAID therapy as well as the prevention of drug induced ulcers. SEARLE

Daktacort
Cream containing hydrocortisone (a topical steroid) and miconazole nitrate (an antifungal and antibacterial agent) for inflamed skin conditions such as eczema and dermatitis in which infection may be a problem. JANSSEN PHARMACEUTICALS

Daktarin Oral Gel
Gel containing miconazole, an antifungal agent. Uses include the treatment and prevention of fungal infections of the throat and gastrointestinal tract.

JANSSEN PHARMACEUTICALS

Daktarin Oral Tablets
Tablets containing miconazole (an antifungal agent). Uses include the treatment and prevention of fungal infections in the throat and gastrointestinal tract.

JANSSEN PHARMACEUTICALS

Dalacin T Topical
Solution and lotion containing clindamycin phosphate (an antibiotic) for the treatment of acne. UPJOHN LTD

Dalmane (Not on the NHS)
Capsules containing flurazepam (a benzodiazepine drug with hypnotic properties) for the short-term treatment of insomnia. ROCHE

Daneral SA Tablets
Tablets containing pheniramine maleate for allergic conditions such as hay fever and other allergies.

HOECHST

Danol
Capsules containing danazol and lactose – uses include the treatment of endometriosis, severe cyclical mastalgia, and for heavy and painful periods.

SANOFI WINTHROP

Daonil Tablets
Tablets containing glibenclamide an anti diabetic drug. HOECHST

Daraprim
Tablets containing pyrimethamine for the prevention and treatment of malaria. WELLCOME

Decadron Tablets
Tablets containing dexamethasone (a corticosteroid). Uses include the treatment of rheumatoid arthritis and Crohn's disease and ulcerative colitis among many others. MERCK SHARP & DOHME LTD

Deca-Durabolin
Injections of nandrolone decanoate for use in osteoporosis in post-menopausal women. ORGANON

Decaserpyl
Tablets containing methoserpidine which produces a slow but sustained reduction in blood pressure. ROUSSEL

Declinax
Tablets containing debrisoquine sulphate for the treatment of high blood pressure. ROCHE

De-Nol
A liquid containing tri-potassium di-citrato bismuthate used as an ulcer-healing agent for the treatment of gastric and duodenal ulcers. BROCADES

De-Noltab
Tablets containing tri-potassium di-citrato bismuthate used as an ulcer-healing agent for the treatment of gastric and duodenal ulcers. BROCADES

Deponit 5 and 10
Patches containing glyceryl trinitrate one of a group of medicines called nitrates used to help prevent angina. SCHWARZ PHARMA

Derbac C Liquid
Liquid containing carbaryl to treat head lice. NAPP

Derbac-M Liquid
Liquid containing malathion for the eradication of head lice, crab lice and their eggs. Treatment of scabies. NAPP

Dermovate Cream
Cream containing clobetasol propionate (a topical steroid), a strong and rapidly effective treatment for inflamed skin conditions such as eczema, dermatitis and psoriasis. GLAXO

Dermovate-NN Cream/ Ointment
Cream or ointment containing clobetasol propionate (a topical steroid), neomycin (an

antibacterial agent) and nystatin (an anticandidal agent), a strong and rapidly effective treatment for inflamed skin conditions such as eczema, dermatitis and psoriasis in which infection may be a problem. GLAXO

Deseril
Tablets containing methysergide maleate (a powerful serotonin antagonist). Serotonin is an enzyme involved in the vascular changes which produce headaches. Uses include the prevention of migraine annd cluster headaches. SANDOZ

Dexa-Rhinaspray
Nasal spray containing tramazoline hydrochloride (a vasoconstrictor) , dexamethasone-21 isonicotinate (a corticosteroid) and neomycin sulphate (an antibiotic) for the treatment of allergic rhinitis.
BOEHRINGER INGELHEIM

Dextropropoxyphene
An analgesic to treat pain.

DHC Continus
Tablets containing dihydrocodeine tartrate in a patented controlled relase system for the relief of chronic severe pain. NAPP

diamorphine linctus
A generic linctus that can be prescribed for use as a cough suppressant.

Dianette
Tablets containing anti-androgen cyproterone acetate and the oestrogen ethinyloestradiol for severe acne. Although Dianette also acts as an oral contraceptive, it is not recommended solely for contraception.
SCHERING HEALTH CARE

Diclomax Retard
Capsules containing diclofenac, a non-steroidal anti-inflammatory analgesic used to treat a number of painful conditions affecting the joints and muscles, for example, rheumatoid arthritis, low back pain, frozen shoulder, tendinitis, sprains, strains and dislocations, gout and after minor surgery. PARKE DAVIS

Didronel PMO
A two component non-hormonal therapy consisting of Didronel tablets containing etidronate disodium and Cacit tablets containing calcium carbonate, for the treatment of established vertebral osteoporosis.
PROCTER & GAMBLE

Difflam
Cream containing benzydamine hydrochloride a topical analgesic and non-steroidal anti-inflammatory agent for sprains and strains etc. 3M HEALTH CARE

Difflam Oral Rinse
A locally acting analgesic and anti-inflammatory containing benzydamine hydrochloride for the relief of painful inflammatory conditions of the mouth and throat. 3M HEALTH CARE

Dihydrocodeine
A narcotic analgesic to relieve pain.

dihydrocodeine elixir
A cough suppressant.

Dimetriose
Capsules containing gestrinone used for the treatment of endometriosis. ROUSSEL

Dimotane La/Tablets/Elixir
Tablets or elixir containing brompheniramine maleate (an antihistamine) for allergic conditions and reactions such as hay fever and urticaria. WYETH

Dimotane Plus LA/Plus/ Plus Paediatric
Tablets or liquid containing brompheniramine maleate (an antihistamine) and pseudoephedrine hydrochloride (a decongestant) for the symptomatic relief of allergic rhinitis. WYETH

Dioctyl
Tablets, solution and paediatric solution containing docusate sodium for constipation. MEDO

Dioctyl Ear Drops
Liquid containing docusate sodium for the softening of ear wax making its removal easier. MEDO

Dioralyte Sachets Plain, Blackcurrant and Citrus
Sachets containing sodium chloride, potassium chloride, glucose and disodium hydrogen citrate for correction of fluid and electrolyte loss in infants, children and adults after diarrhoea Effervescent tablets also available. RHONE-POULENC RORER

Diprobase
Emollient cream or ointment containing liquid paraffin and white soft paraffin to soothe, moisturise and protect dry skin conditions. They can also be used as a medium for topical steroids. SCHERING-PLOUGH

Diprobath
Bath emollient containing light liquid paraffin and isopropyl myristate. It deposits a thin film of oil over the skin and slows down moisture loss so is useful in dry skin conditions. SCHERING-PLOUGH

Diprosalic
Ointment or scalp application containing betamethasone (a corticosteroid) and salicylic acid (to soften and loosen the skin) for the treatment of chronic lichenified eczema, lichen planus, lichen simplex, non bullous ichthyosiform erythroderma – severe dry skin condition with inflammation. It's also effective in psoriasis of the scalp and chronic plaque psoriasis of the hands and feet but excluding widespread plaque psoriasis. SCHERING-PLOUGH

Disalcid
Analgesic capsules containing salsalate for the treatment of arthritis, bursitis, fibrositis etc. 3M HEALTH CARE

Disipal
Tablets containing orphenadrine hydrochloride for the treatment of all forms of Parkinson's disease, including drug-induced. BROCADES

Disprol Paediatric
A suspension containing paracetamol for the treatment of mild to moderate pain in children. RECKITT & COLMAN

Diprosone
Cream, ointment or lotion containing betamethasone (a corticosteroid) for eczema and dermatitis. The lotion is a slightly gelled solution also containing isopropyl alcohol, which has antibacterial activity. It's formulated to spread without sticking to hair. SCHERING-PLOUGH

Dithrocream
Cream containing dithranol for psoriasis including psoriasis of the scalp. DERMAL

Dithrolan
Ointment containing dithranol and salicylic acid for the treatment of quiescent psoriasis. DERMAL

Diurexan
Tablets containing xipamide (a diuretic), an antihypertensive agent for high blood pressure and fluid retention. ASTA MEDICA

Dixarit
Tablets containing clonidine hydrochloride (which counteracts the body's overreacting nerve and

chemical system) for the prevention of migraine and the management of vasomotor conditions commonly associated with the menopause and characterised by flushing. BOEHRINGER INGELHEIM

Dolobid and Dolobid 500
Tablets containing diflunisal for the relief of pain and for the relief of pain and inflammation in osteoarthritis and rheumatoid arthritis; and painful periods. THOMAS MORSON PHARMACEUTICALS

Dramamine
Antihistamine tablet containing dimenhydrinate for travel sickness, vertigo, nausea and vomiting associated with Menière's disease and other labyrinthine disorders. SEARLE

Duovent
Inhaler containing fenoterol hydrobromide and ipratropium bromide (drugs with bronchodilator properties) for the treatment of reversible airways obstruction as in bronchial asthma, bronchitis and emphysema. BOEHRINGER INGELHEIM

Duphaston
Tablets containing dydrogesterone (a progestogen). Uses include counteracting the effects of unopposed oestrogen in hormone replacement therapy; premenstrual syndrome; endometriosis; painful periods. DUPHAR

Durabolin
Injections of nandrolone phenylpropionate for use in osteoporosis in post-menopausal women. ORGANON

Efamast
Capsules containing gamolenic acid provided by evening primrose oil for the symptomatic relief of premenstrual breast pain (cyclical mastalgia) and non-cyclical mastalgia. SEARLE

Efalith Ointment
Ointment containing lithium succinate and zinc sulphate for the treatment of seborrhoeic dermatitis. SEARLE

Efcortelan Cream/ Ointment
Cream or ointment containing hydrocortisone (a topical steroid) – a mild treatment for inflamed skin conditions such as eczema and dermatitis. GLAXO

Eldepryl
Tablets containing selegiline hydrochloride for the

treatment of Parkinson's disease.

BRITANNIA PHARMACEUTICALS LTD

Electrolade

Oral replacement therapy for electrolyte and fluid loss as a result of diarrhoea or other feverish illnesses. Sachets contain sodium chloride, potassium chloride, sodium bicarbonate and glucose.

ROCHE NICHOLAS

Elocon

Ointment, lotion or smooth cream containing mometasone furoate (a topical corticosteroid) for the treatment of psoriasis (excluding widespread plaque psoriasis) and atopic dermatitis. It's also used for the treatment of scalp psoriasis and seborrhoeic dermatitis. SCHERING-PLOUGH

Eltroxin

Tablets containing thyroxine used to treat an underactive thyroid gland. EVANS MEDICAL

Emcor/Emcor LS

Tablets containing bisoprolol fumarate (a beta-blocker) for the management of high blood pressure and angina.

MERCK

Emflex

Capsules containing acemetacin (a non-steroidal anti-inflammatory drug) for rheumatoid arthritis, osteoarthritis and post-operative pain and inflammation. MERCK

Epanutin

Capsules, suspension and chewable tablets containing phenytoin (an anticonvulsant) to treat epilepsy. PARKE DAVIS

ephedrine nasal drops

Decongestant nasal drops.

Epilim

Tablets, syrup or liquid containing sodium valproate one of a group of medicines called anticonvulsant or anti-epileptic agents used to treat epilepsy. SANOFI WINTHROP

Epogam/Epogam Paediatric

Capsules containing gamolenic acid provided by evening primrose oil for the symptomatic relief of eczema.

SEARLE

Equagesic (Not on the NHS)

Tablets containing ethoheptazine citrate, meprobamate and aspirin – an analgesic with muscle-relaxant properties for the short-term symptomatic treatment of pain in musculo-skeletal disorders. WYETH

Erymax

Capsules containing the antibiotic erythromycin for the treatment of upper and lower respiratory tract infections of mild to moderate severity; skin and soft tissue infections including pustular acne. PARKE DAVIS

Erythroped A, Erythroped A Sachet, Erythroped PI SF, SF, PI SF Sachet and SF Sachet

Tablets, suspension and sachets of eryhromycin used to treat a wide variety of infections, tonsillitis, sinusitis, boils, etc. ABBOTT LABORATORIES

Esidrex

Tablets containing hydrochlorothiazide used as a diuretic and to treat high blood pressure. CIBA

Estracombi

HRT patches of oestrogen and also oestrogen and progestogen for symptoms of the menopause and for the prevention of osteoporosis. CIBA

Estraderm TTS

HRT patches of oestrogen for symptoms of the menopause and prevention of osteoporosis. CIBA

Estrapak 50

HRT patches containing oestrogen and tablets containing progestogen to relieve symptoms of the menopause and for the prevention of osteoporosis. CIBA

Euglucon

Tablets containing glibenclamide – an oral hypoglycaemic agent which reduces the concentration of glucose in the blood. For the treatment of maturity-onset diabetes which is not adequately controlled by dietary measures alone. ROUSSEL

Eugynon 30

Combined oestrogen-progestogen oral contraceptive containing levonorgestrel and ethinyloestradiol. SCHERING

Eumovate Cream/Ointment

Cream or ointment containing clobetasone butyrate (a topical steroid) – a rapidly effective treatment for inflamed skin conditions such as eczema, dermatitis and psoriasis. GLAXO

Eurax
Cream containing crotamiton. Uses include the treatment of scabies and the symptomatic relief of pruritus of varying origins. ZYMA

Eurax Hydrocortisone
Cream containing crotamiton and hydrocortisone for eczema and dermatitis. ZYMA

Exelderm Cream
A cream containing sulconazole nitrate used as an anti-fungal agent for athlete's foot, thrush and other fungal infections of the skin. ICI

Exirel
Metered inhaler or capsules providing pirbuterol acetate for asthma and bronchitis. 3M HEALTH CARE

Fansidar
Tablets containing sulfadoxine and pyrimethamine for the treatment and prevention of malaria. ROCHE

Faverin
Tablets containing fluvoxamine maleate (an anti-depressant) for the symptoms of depression. DUPHAR

Femodene
Combined oestrogen progestogen oral contraceptive containing gestodene and ethinyloestradiol. SCHERING

Femodene ED
Combined oestrogen-progestogen oral contraceptive containing gestodene and ethinyloestradiol. SCHERING

Femulen
A progestogen-only oral contraceptive (the mini-pill) containing ethynodiol diacetate. GOLD CROSS

fenoprofen
An anti-inflammatory non-narcotic analgesic for the treatment of rheumatoid arthritis, oesteoarthritis and to lower fever.

Fergon
Tablets containing ferrous gluconate for the treatment and prevention of uncomplic ated iron deficiency anaemia. SANOFI WINTHROP

Ferrocontin Continus Tablets
Tablets containing ferrous glycine sulphate for the treatment and prevention of iron deficiency anaemia. ASTA MEDICA

Ferrocontin Folic Continus
Tablets containing ferrous glycine sulphate and folic acid for the prophylaxis of iron and folic acid deficiencies during pregnancy. ASTA MEDICA

Ferrograd Folic
Tablets containing dried ferrous sulphate and folic acid for the prevention and treatment of iron-deficiency anaemia of pregnancy. ABBOTT

Ferromyn Elixir
Elixir containing ferrous succinate for the prevention and treatment of iron-deficiency anaemias. WELLCOME

Fertiral
An anti infertility drug containing gonadorelin.
HOECHST

Flamazine Cream
Cream containing silver sulphadiazine (an antibacterial agent) for the prevention and treatment of infection in burn wounds.
SMITH & NEPHEW

Flexin
Tablets containing indomethacin a non-steroidal anti-inflammatory agent used to treat arthritis, low back pain, and inflammatory disorders such as bursitis. NAPP

Flixonase
Nasal spray containing fluticasone propionate for the prevention and treatment of seasonal allergic rhinitis.
ALLEN & HANBURYS

Flixotide Diskhaler
Dishaler containing fluticasone propionate – preventive treatment for asthma. ALLEN & HANBURYS

Floxapen
Capsules or syrup containing flucloxacillin, an antibiotic used to treat skin and soft tissue infections and respiratory tract infections among others. BEECHAM RESEARCH

Folicin
Tablets containing dried ferrous sulphate, copper sulphate, manganese sulphate and folic acid for the prevention and treatment of anaemia of pregnancy.
PAINES & BYRNE

Fortagesic (Not on the NHS)
Compound analgesic tablets containing pentazocine and paracetamol for the relief of moderate pain associated with musculoskeletal disorders or injuries, such as bursitis, sprains and strains and arthritis. SANOFI WINTHROP

Franol
Tablets containing theophylline and ephedrine hydrochloride for the management of bronchospasm in reversible airway obstruction associated with stable asthma or chronic bronchitis. SANOFI WINTHROP

Franol Plus
Tablets containing theophylline and ephedrine sulphate for the management of bronchospasm in reversible airway-obstruction associated with stable asthma or chronic bronchitis. SANOFI WINTHROP

Frisium (Not on the NHS)
An anti-epileptic agent and anxiolytic containing clobazam (a benzodiazepine) for the short-term relief (two to four weeks) of anxiety and as an adjunctive therapy in epilepsy. HOECHST

Frusene
Tablets containing frusemide and triamterene for use as a potassium conserving diuretic to treat fluid retention caused by heart and hepatic oedema, i.e. heart or liver failure. FISONS

Fulcin, Fulcin Oral Suspension
Antibiotic containing griseofulvin for the treatment of ringworm and for the treatment of fungal infections of the skin, hair and nails when topical therapy has failed or is considered inappropriate. ICI

Fungilin
Lozenges, suspension and tablets containing antifungal antibiotic amphotericin. Uses include oral thrush, and intestinal thrush and the suppression of the intestinal reservoir of *candida albicans* which may precipitate cutaneous or vaginal candidosis normally known as thrush of the skin or vagina. SQUIBB

Furadantin
Tablets or suspension containning nitrofurantoin (an antibiotic) for treatment and prevention of urinary tract infections. PROCTER & GAMBLE

Fybogel and Fybogel Orange
Granules of ispaghula husk for the treatment of constipation and for patients who need a high fibre diet. RECKITT & COLMAN

Fybogel Mebeverine
Granules containing ispaghula husk and mebeverine hydrochloride (which can help relax muscle

spasm) for the treatment of abdominal pain and bowel dysfunction associated with irritable bowel syndrome and other gastrointestinal diseases. RECKITT & COLMAN

Galenamet
Tablets containing cimetidine (an H2 antagonist) for ulcer disease and heartburn.
GALEN LTD

Galcodine
Linctus and paediatric linctus containing codeine phosphate (a cough suppressant) for the relief of unproductive dry cough in adults and children.
GALEN LTD

Galenamox
Capsules or suspension of amoxycillin (an antibiotic). Uses include dental infections; upper respiratory tract infections; bronchitis, pneumonia; cystitis; gynaecological infections; gonorrhoea. GALEN LTD

Galenphol
Medicines containing pholcodine (a cough suppressant) for the relief of unproductive dry coughs.
GALEN LTD

Galfloxin
Capsules containing flucloxacillin (an antibiotic). Uses include respiratory tract infections, infected skin and soft tissue injuries, mengingitis, urinary tract infections. GALEN LTD

Galpseud Linctus/Tablets
Linctus or tablets containing pseudoephedrine hydrochloride (a decongestant) for the relief of nasal, sinus and upper respiratory congestion.
GALEN LTD

Galpseud Plus Linctus
Linctus containing pseudoephedrine hydrochloride(a decongestant) and chlorpheniramine maleate (an antihistamine) for the relief of allergic rhinitis. GALEN LTD

Gamanil
Tablets containing lofepramine hydrochloride for treating the symptoms of depression. MERCK

Gastrobid Continus
Tablets containing metoclopramide hydrochloride to restore normal coordination and tone to the upper digestive tract.
NAPP

Gastron
Tablets containing alginic acid, dried aluminium

hydroxide, sodium bicarbonate and magnesium trisilicate to alleviate heartburn. SANOFI WINTHROP

Gaviscon (Liquid) and Gaviscon Tablets
A suspension containing sodium alginate, sodium bicarbonate and calcium carbonate. Tablets containing alginic acid, magnesium trisilicate, dried aluminium hydroxide and sodium bicarbonate for heartburn, including heartburn of pregnancy, dyspepsia associated with gastric reflux, hiatus hernia, and problems associated with gastric reflux.
RECKITT & COLMAN

Geangin
Tablets containing verapamil hydrochloride (a calcium channel blocker) for the treatment and prevention of angina; high blood pressure and treatment and prevention of supraventricular tachycardia – an abnormally rapid heartbeat, initiated from the top part of the heart.
CUSI (UK) LTD

Genticin Eye/Ear Drops
Drops containing gentamicin (an antibiotic) for superficial infections of the eye or ear – e.g. conjunctivitis and otitis externa – and for the prevention against infection in trauma of the eye or ear.
ROCHE NICHOLAS

Genticin Eye Ointment
Eye ointment containing gentamicin (an antibiotic) useful in external bacterial infections of the eye particularly conjunctivitis, blepharitis, styes, corneal ulcers and as a preventive measure in trauma.
ROCHE NICHOLAS

Genticin Ointment
Ointment containing gentamicin sulphate (an antibiotic) for bacterial skin infections and infected wounds and ulcers.
ROCHE NICHOLAS

Gentisone HC Cream/ Ointment
Cream or ointment containing hydrocortisone acetate and gentamicin sulphate (an antibiotic) for infective eczemas, infective contact dermatitis, inflammation of the external ear and infected pruritis. ROCHE NICHOLAS

Gentisone HC Ear Drops
Antibiotic and corticosteroid ear drops containing gentamicin sulphate and hydrocortisone acetate. Uses include bacterial infections of the ear, as well as eczema

and infection of the outer ear. ROCHE NICHOLAS

Glurenorm

Tablets containing gliquidone for the treatment of non-insulin dependent diabetes mellitus which does not respond adequately to dietary measures. SANOFI WINTHROP

Glytrin Spray

Aerosol providing glyceryl trinitrate for the treatment and prevention of angina. SANOFI WINTHROP

Guarina

Sachets of guar gum as an adjunct in the treatment of diabetes mellitus. NORGINE

Gyno-Daktarin

Cream containing miconazole nitrate (an anti-fungal agent). Uses include the treatment of thrush. JANSSEN

Hamarin

Tablets containing allopurinol for gout and for the prevention of uric acid and calcium oxylate stones. ROCHE NICHOLAS

Harmogen

Oestrogen HRT tablets for symptoms of the menopause and prevention of oesteoporosis. ABBOTT

Herpid

Solution containing idoxuridine (an antiviral agent) for herpes (including cold sores) and shingles. BOEHRINGER INGELHEIM

Hewletts Cream

A cream containing zinc oxide and lanolin for use as a mild aseptic and astringent in the care of mildly inflamed skin such as nappy rash and sore hands. BIOGLAN

Hiprex

Tablets containing methenamine hippurate used in the prevention and treatment of urinary tract infections. 3M HEALTH CARE

Hirudoid

Cream or gel containing the organo-heparinoid 'Luitpold' for the soothing relief of superficial bruising and haematoma. Also for the treatment of superficial thrombophlebitis. PANPHARMA

Hismanal

Tablets containing astemizole, a long-acting antihistamine for allergic rhinitis and conjunctivitis and other conditions normally responsive to antihistamines, including allergic skin reactions (urticaria). JANSSEN

Hormonin

HRT oestrogen tablets for menopausal symptoms and the prevention of oesteoporosis. SHIRE

Hydrocal

Hydrocortisone acetate in a calamine cream base for the treatment of mild eczema, allergic dermatitis and nappy rash. BIOGLAN

Hydrocortisyl skin cream and ointment

Cream and ointment containing micronised hydrocortisone for eczema and dermatitis of all types, intertrigo and insect bite reactions. ROUSSEL

Hydromet

Tablets containing methyldopa and hydrochlorothiazide, two antihypertensive agents for the treatment of high blood pressure. MERCK SHARP & DOHME LTD

Hydrosaluric

Tablets containing hydrochlorothiazide (a diuretic and antihypertensive agent) for fluid retention associated with congestive heart failure, premenstrual tension and renal dysfunction. Also for high blood pressure.

MERCK SHARP & DOHME LTD

Hygroton

Tablets containing chlorthalidone – a diuretic for the treatment of mild to moderate high blood pressure and fluid retention. GEIGY

Hygroton K

Tablets containing chlorthalidone (a diuretic) and potassium chloride for mild to moderate high blood pressure and fluid retention where a potassium supplement is needed. GEIGY

Hytrin

Anti-hypertensive tablets containing terazosin used to treat mild to moderate high blood pressure.

ABBOTT LABORATORIES

Imdur

Tablets containing isosorbide mononitrate for the prevention of angina. ASTRA

Imigran Tablets/ Autoinjector

Tablets or autoinjector containing sumatriptan to treat migraine. GLAXO

Imodium

Capsules or syrup containing loperamide hydrochloride for the symptomatic treatment of diarrhoea. JANSSEN

Imperacin Tablets
Tablets containing oxytetracycline dihydrate, a broad spectrum antibiotic. ICI

Imunovir
Tablets containing inosine pranobex (an anti-viral agent) for the management of infections due to herpes simplex virus. LEO

Inderal
Tablets containing propranolol (a beta blocker) for high blood pressure, angina, anxiety, migraine and some disorders of heart rhythm. ICI PHARMACEUTICALS

Inderal LA/Half-Inderal LA
Capsules containing propranolol hydrochloride (a beta-blocker). Uses include the management of angina, anxiety symptoms, the prevention of migraine and in the control of high blood pressure. ICI PHARMACEUTICALS

Inderetic
Capsules containing propranolol hydrochloride (a beta-blocker) and bendrofluazide (a diuretic) for the management of high blood pressure.
ICI PHARMACEUTICALS

Inderex
A combination of two treatments, propranolol (a beta blocker) and bendrofluazide (a diuretic) for high blood pressure.
ICI PHARMACEUTICALS

Indocid
Capsules, suspension and suppositories containing indomethacin a non-steroidal anti-inflammatory agent used in the treatment of arthritis and painful periods.
THOMAS MORSON PHARMACEUTICALS

Infacol
An antiflatulent containing activated dimethicone for the relief of griping pain, colic or wind due to swallowed air.
PHARMAX

Infant Gaviscon
Powder containing sodium alginate, magnesium alginate and dried aluminium hydroxide for gastric regurgitation, gastro-oesophageal reflux and reflux associated with hiatus hernia in infants and young children.
RECKITT & COLMAN

Innozide
Tablets containing enalapril maleate (an angiotensin-converting enzyme inhibitor) – a medicine which inhibits an enzyme to achieve its effect,

and hydrochlorothiazide (a diuretic) for the treatement of mild to moderate hypertension.

MERCK SHARP & DOHME LTD

Innovace

Tablets containing enalapril maleate for the treatment of high blood pressure and heart failure. MERCK SHARP & DOHME LTD

Intal

Sodium cromoglycate available as Intal spincaps for use in the Intal Spinhaler, Intal Compound spincaps for use in the Intal spinhaler, Intal Inhaler, Intal Nebuliser Solution and Intal Fisonair – for the preventive treatment of bronchial asthma. FISONS

Intralgin

Rub containing benzocaine and salicylamide for the relief of muscle pain. 3M HEALTH CARE

Ionax Scrub

A gel containing polyethylene granules, benzalkonium chloride, macrogol (4) lauryl ether, macrogol (23) lauryl ether and alcohol for use as an abradant cleanser for the control and hygiene of acne.

GALDERMA (UK) LTD

Ionil T shampoo

A shampoo with salicylic acid, benzalkonium chloride and coal tar solution for seborrhoeic dermatitis and psoriasis of the scalp.

GALDERMA (UK) LTD

Ismelin

Tablets containing guanethidine – one of the group of medicines called anti-hypertensives which are used to reduce high blood pressure. CIBA

isoaminile linctus

Linctus used to treat dry, persistent coughs.

Isogel

A natural-fibre drink containing dried ispaghula husk, a natural source of non-starch carbohydrate fibre, the fibre type considered to be the most suitable means of increasing faecal bulk. Isogel is both effective as a laxative and helpful in the control of diarrhoea associated with disorders such as irritable bowel syndrome, making it an ideal preparation for promoting natural bowel regularity. It's also useful in the management of colostomies.

CHARWELL PHARMACEUTICALS

Junifen

Liquid containing ibuprofen for mild to moderate pain and

fever in children over one year old. BOOTS

Kalspare
Tablets containing chlorthalidone and triamterene. Kalspare is a potassium-sparing diuretic and antihypertensive for the management of mild to moderate high blood pressure and fluid retention. CUSI (UK) LTD

Kalspare LS
Tablets containing chlorthalidone and triamterene. Kalspare LS is a potassium sparing diuretic for the treatment of mild to moderate high blood pressures. CUSI (UK) LTD

Kalten
Capsules containing atenolol (a beta-blocker), hydrochlorothiazide (a diuretic) and amiloride hydrochloride (a diuretic used primarily for its potassium-conserving effects) for the management of high blood pressure. STUART PHARMACEUTICALS

Kamillosan
Ointment containing chamomile extracts in a base containing lanolin for the prevention and treatment of sore nipples in nursing mothers, nappy rash and chapped hands. NORGINE

Kemadrin
Tablets or injection containing procyclidine hydrochloride for all forms of Parkinson's disease. WELLCOME

Klaricid
Tablets containing clarithromycin (an antibiotic which is a semi-synthetic derivative of erythromycin A). Uses include treatment of upper and lower respiratory tract infections; skin and soft tissue infections. Also available as Klaricid Paediatric Suspension which is also used to treat ear infections. ABBOTT LABORATORIES

Kolanticon Gel
Suspension containing dicyclomine hydrochloride, dried aluminium hydroxide gel, light magnesium oxide, and simethicone, an antacid antiflatulent anti-spasmodic demulcent for the treatment and prevention of peptic ulcer, dyspepsia and for relief in oesophagitis, hiatus hernia, gastritis. MARION MERRELL DOW

lactitol
A laxative used for constipation.

lactulose solution BP
A solution of lactulose used to treat constipation.

Lamictal
Antiepileptic drug containing lamotrigine. WELLCOME

Lamisil Cream
Cream containing terbinafine hydrochloride for fungal skin infections. SANDOZ

Lamisil Tablets
Tablets containing terbinafine hydrochloride (an anti-fungal agent) for the treatment of ringworm and other fungal skin infections where oral therapy is considered appropriate due to the site, severity or extent of the infection. SANDOZ

Lariam
Tablets containing mefloquine hydrochloride therapy for prevention of malaria. ROCHE

Lasikal Tablets
Tablets containing frusemide and potassium chloride – a short-acting diuretic and a slow-release potassium supplement for the treatment of fluid retention in patients who need potassium supplementation. HOECHST

Lasipressin
Tablets containing frusemide and penbutolol sulphate for the management of high blood pressure. HOECHST

Lasix Tablets
Tablets containing frusemide, a diuretic. HOECHST

Lasix + K Combination Pack
Tablets containing frusemide (a diuretic) and potassium chloride tablets. HOECHST

Lasix Paediatric Liquid
Liquid containing frusemide (a diuretic) for fluid retention in children. It may be used in elderly patients or those unable to take solid oral dose forms of Lasix. HOECHST

Lasma
Tablets containing theophylline for the treatment and prophylaxis of bronchospasm associated with asthma, emphysema and bronchitis. PHARMAX

Lasonil
An ointment for bruises, sprains, piles and soft-tissue injuries. Contains heparinoid, an anti-inflammatory agent, and hyaluronidase, an enzyme which makes tissue more permeable. BAYER

Lentizol

Capsules containing amitriptyline hydrochloride for the symptoms of depression especially where sedation is needed. PARKE DAVIS

Lexotan (Not on the NHS)

Tablets containing bromazepam for the short-term treatment of anxiety.

ROCHE

Librium (Generic on the NHS)

Capsules and tablets containing chlordiazepoxide for the short-term treatment of anxiety, symptomatic relief of acute alcohol withdrawal.

ROCHE

Limbitrol

Capsules containing chlordiazepoxide and amitriptyline hydrochloride for the treatment of depression with associated anxiety. ROCHE

Lingraine

Tablets containing ergotamine tartrate for the relief of migraine.

SANOFI WINTHROP

Lipobase

An emollient cream for dry skin conditions which can also be used as a medium for other medicines. BROCADES

Lipantil

Capsules containing fenofibrate for high cholesterol. FOURNIER

Lipostat

Tablets containing pravastatin sodium for high cholesterol. SQUIBB

Livial

HRT tablets containing tibolone – single molecule with oestrogen and progestogen activities.

ORGANON

Loceryl

Cream or nail lacquer containing amorolfine (a topical antimycotic) for fungal skin infections. ROCHE

Locoid C Cream/Ointment

Cream containing hydrocortisone and chlorquinaldol (an antibacterial and antifungal agent) for eczema, dermatitis and psoriasis where secondary bacterial or fungal infection is present or needs to be prevented. BROCADES

Locoid Cream/Ointment

Cream or ointment containing hydrocortisone for eczema and dermatitis; psoriasis (excluding widespread plaque psoriasis). BROCADES

Locoid Lipocream
Cream containing hydrocortisone for eczema, dermatitis and psoriasis.
BROCADES

Locoid Scalp Lotion
Lotion for scalp conditions including seborrhoea with or without an associated severe dandruff and psoriasis of the scalp. BROCADES

Locorten-Vioform Ear Drops
Antibacterial, antifungal and anti-inflammatory drops containing clioquinol and flumethasone pivalate for the treatment of inflammatory conditions of the external ear where a secondary infection is suspected. ZYMA

Lodine
Capsules or tablets containing etodolac – a non-steroidal anti-inflammatory drug – for acute or long-term use in rheumatoid arthrits and osteoarthritis. WYETH

Loestrin
Combined contraceptive pill containing norethisterone acetate and ethinyloestradiol.
PARKE DAVIS

Logynon/Logynon Ed
Combined oestrogen-progestogen oral contraceptives containing ethinyloestradiol and levonorgestrel. SCHERING

Lomotil Tablets/Liquid
Tablets or liquid containing diphenoxylate hydrochloride and atropine sulphate for diarrhoea, in some cases relief of symptoms in chronic mild ulcerative colitis and for the control of stool formation after colostomy or ileostomy.
GOLD CROSS

Lopid
Capsules or tablets containing gemfibrozil for high cholesterol. PARKE-DAVIS

loprazolam tablets
Loprazalam tablets for the short-term treatment of insomnia including difficulty in falling asleep and frequent waking at night.

Lopresor
Tablets containing metoprolol tartrate (a beta-blocker). Uses include treatment of high blood pressure, angina and abnormal heart rhythm, and prevention of migraine. GEIGY

Lopresor SR
Tablets containing metoprolol tartrate (a beta-blocker). Used in the treatment of high blood pressure, angina and for the prevention of migraine. GEIGY

Lopresoretic
Tablets containing metoprolol tartrate (a beta-blocker) and chlorthalidone (a diuretic) for mild and moderate high blood pressure. GEIGY

Lorazepam Tablets
Tablets containing lorazepam (a benzodiazepine) for the short term treatment of anxiety and similar uses to Ativan. WYETH

lormetazepam tablets
Tablets containing lormetazepam for the short term treatment of insomnia.

Losec
Capsules containing omeprazole. Uses include the treatment of reflux oesophagitis and the treatment of duodenal and benign gastric ulcers. ASTRA

Lotriderm Cream
Cream containing betamethasone (a corticosteroid) and clotrimazole (an anti-fungal agent) for the short-term treatment of fungal skin infections where there's inflammation. SCHERING-PLOUGH

Ludiomil
Tablets containing maprotiline (an antidepressant) used to treat depression. CIBA

Lurselle
Tablets containing probucol for the treatment of high cholesterol. MARION MERRELL DOW

Lyclear Creme Rinse
Rinse containing permethrin and isopropanol for the treatment of head lice.
WELLCOME

Lyclear Dermal Cream
Cream containing permethrin for the treatment of scabies.
WELLCOME

Maalox Suspension and Tablets
Suspension or tablets containing dried aluminium hydroxide gel and magnesium hydroxide used as antacid therapy for the relief of gastritis, dyspepsia and gastric hyperacidity.
RHONE-POULENC RORER

Maalox TC Suspension and Tablets
Suspension or tablets containing dried aluminium hydroxide and magnesium hydroxide for the management of heartburn, gastric hyperacidity and gastritis; the treatment and prevention of duodenal ulcer and the management of the

symptoms of peptic ulceration. RHONE-POULENC RORER

MacroBID
Capsules containing nitrofurantoin (an antibiotic) uses include the treatment of urinary tract infections. PROCTER & GAMBLE

Macrodantin Capsules
Capsules of nitrofurantoin, an antibiotic, for the treatment and prevention of urinary tract infections. PROCTER & GAMBLE

Madopar
Capsules or dispersible tablets containing levodopa for the treatment of Parkinson's disease. ROCHE

Madopar CR
Capsules containing levodopa and benserazide for Parkinson's disease. ROCHE

magnesium hydroxide
An antacid that also has laxative properties.

magnesium trisilicate
A long-acting antacid.

Maloprim
Tablets containing pyrimethamine and dapsone for the prevention and treatment of malaria. WELLCOME

Manerix Tablets
Tablets containing moclobemide used to treat depression. ROCHE

Manevac
Granules containing ispaghula and senna for symptoms of constipation. GALEN LTD

Marvelon
Combined oral contraceptive containing desogestrel and ethinyloestradiol. ORGANON

Masnoderm Cream
Cream containing clotrimazole (an antifungal agent) for the treatment of skin infections including ringworm, athlete's foot, intertrigo, fungal nappy rash and thrush. CUSI

Medihaler
Inhalation therapy containing isoprenaline (a bronchodilator) for asthma and bronchitis. 3M HEALTH CARE

Medihaler Ergotamine
Aerosol containing ergotamine tartrate for rapid relief of migraine. 3M HEALTH CARE

Medrone Tablets
Tablets containing methylprednisolone a powerful corticosteroid. Uses include Crohn's disease,

bronchial asthma, rheumatoid arthritis, allergies. UPJOHN LTD

Menzol
Tablets containing norethisterone (a progestogen) for premenstrual syndrome, painful periods and menorrhagia (heavy periods). SCHWARZ PHARMA

Merbentyl Syrup, Merbentyl Tablets and 20 Tablets
Syrup and tablets containing dicyclomine hydrochloride (an antispasmodic agent) for the treatment of functional conditions involving smooth muscle spasm of the gastro-intestinal tract. The commonest of these is irritable colon. MARION MERRELL DOW

Mercilon
Combined oral contraceptive containing desogestrel and ethinyloestradiol. ORGANON

Metenix 5 Tablets
Tablets containing metolazone, a diuretic. Uses include the treatment of high blood pressure. HOECHST

Meterfolic
Tablets containing ferrous fumarate and folic acid for the prevention of iron and folic acid deficiencies in pregnancy. SINCLAIR PHARMACEUTICALS

methadone linctus
A cough suppressant.

Metosyn FapG Cream and Ointment
Cream and ointment containing fluocinonide (a topical steroid) for a wide variety of skin conditions including eczema and dermatitis, and psoriasis. STUART PHARMACEUTICALS

Metosyn Scalp Lotion
Scalp lotion containing fluocinonide (a topical steroid) used to treat several conditions of the scalp including psoriasis, and severe types of dandruff. STUART PHARMACEUTICALS

Microgynon 30
Combined oestrogen-progestogen oral contraceptive containing levonorgestrel and ethinyloestradiol. SCHERING

Micronor
Progestogen only oral contraceptive containing norethisterone. ORTHO

Microval
Mini pill containing levonorgestrel. WYETH

Mictral
Granules containing nalidixic acid, sodium citrate, citric acid, and sodium bicarbonate for the treatment of cystitis and lower urinary tract infections. SANOFI WINTHROP

Midamor
Tablets containing amiloride hydrochloride used as a diuretic.
THOMAS MORSON PHARMACEUTICALS

Midrid
Capsules containing isometheptene mucate and paracetamol for the treatment of migraine. SHIRE

Migraleve
Tablets to relieve migraine headache, nausea and vomiting. Pack contains eight pink and four yellow tablets. Pink tablets contain the pain-relievers paracetamol and codeine phosphate and the antihistamine buclizine hydrochloride. Yellow tablets do not contain buclizine hydrochloride.
CHARWELL PHARMACEUTICALS

Migravess/Migravess Forte
Anti-emetic and analgesic tablets containing metoclopramide monohydrochloride, aspirin, sodium bicarbonate, and citric acid for the rapid symptomatic relief of headache and nausea associated with migraine.
BAYER

Migril
Tablets containing ergotamine tartrate, cyclizine hydrochloride and caffeine for the relief of acute migraine attack. WELLCOME

Mildison Lipocream
Cream containing hydrocortisone for eczema and dermatitis and insect bite reactions. BROCADES

Minims Chloramphenicol
Eye drops containing chloramphenicol a topical antibacterial for the treatment of superficial eye infections.
SMITH & NEPHEW

Minims Gentamicin Sulphate
Eye drops containing gentamicin sulphate a broad spectrum antibiotic for the treatment of eye infections.
SMITH & NEPHEW

Minims Neomycin Sulphate
Eye drops containing neomycin sulphate (an antibiotic) for the treatment of bacterial eye infections.
SMITH & NEPHEW

Mintec Capsules
Capsules containing peppermint oil for the treatment of discomfort and pain and distension associated with the irritable bowel or spastic colon syndrome. SMITH KLINE AND FRENCH

Minulet
Combined oestrogen-progestogen contraceptive pill containing ethinyloestradiol and gestodene. WYETH

Miraxid
Antibiotic tablets, suspension containing pivampicillin and pivmecillinam hydrochloride. Uses include acute bronchitis, otitis media, sinusitis, tonsillitis, tracheitis, laryngitis, pharyngitis and urinary tract infections. FISONS

Mobiflex
Tablets or granules containing tenoxicam (a non-steroidal anti-inflammatory drug) for the relief of pain and inflammation in osteoarthrits and rheumatoid arthritis. Also for the short-term management of acute musculoskeletal disorders including strains, sprains and other soft-tissue injuries.
ROCHE

Modrasone
Cream or ointment containing alclometasone dipropionate (a corticosteroid) for inflammatory skin conditions such as eczema and dermatitis. SCHERING-PLOUGH

Moducren
Tablets containing hydrochlorothiazide, amiloride hydrochloride and timolol maleate used in the treatment of mild to moderate high blood pressure.
THOMAS MORSON PHARMACEUTICALS

Mogadon (Generic on the NHS)
Tablets or capsules containing nitrazepam for the short-term treatment of insomnia. ROCHE

Molipaxin
Tablets, capsules or liquid containing trazodone hydrochloride as a powerful anti-depressant. It also has anxiety reducing activity.
ROUSSEL

Monit/Monit LS Tablets
Contain isosorbide mononitrate (a vasodilator) to help prevent an attack of chest pain (angina).
STUART PHARMACEUTICALS

Monotrim
Tablets containing trimethoprim (an

antibacterial drug). Uses include the treatment of urinary and respiratory tract infections. DUPHAR

Morhulin
Cod-liver oil and zinc oxide for nappy rash. NAPP

Morsep
An antiseptic cream containing cetrimide (an active antiseptic which helps fight infection) and vitamin A which is known to have healing properties. Ideal for the treatment of sore nipples, nappy rash, minor burns and scalds. NAPP

Motilium
Tablets containing domperidone maleate for nausea and vomiting. SANOFI WINTHROP

Motrin
Tablets containing ibuprofen for the relief of the signs and symptoms of arthritis, also for low back pain, sprains and strains etc. UPJOHN LTD

Movelat
Rubefacient cream and gel containing mucopoly-saccharide polysulphate and salicylic acid for the relief of symptoms associated with painful inflammatory conditions of the musculo-skeletal system, including traumatic conditions such as sprains and strains. PANPHARMA

Mucaine
Suspension containing local anaesthetic oxethazaine and antacids magnesium hydroxide, aluminium hydroxide mixture for the symptomatic treatment of oesophagitis whatever its cause including the heartburn of late pregnancy. WYETH

Mucogel
Antacid suspension containing aluminium hydroxide and magnesium hydroxide for the treatment of indigestion, heartburn, antacid therapy in gastric and duodenal ulcer, gastritis, and symptoms associated with hiatus hernia. PHARMAX

Mycardol
Tablets containing pentaerythritol tetranitrate for the symptomatic treatment of angina. SANOFI WINTHROP

Myocrisin
Ampoules for injection containing sodium aurothiomalate for the management of rheumatoid arthritis and progressive juvenile chronic arthritis. RHONE-POULENC RORER

Mysoline

Tablets containing primidone which helps prevent epileptic fits. Sometimes it's used to control severe shaking attacks in patients who aren't epileptic. ICI PHARMACEUTICALS

Nalcrom

Nalcrom is a presentation of sodium cromoglycate for oral use in the treatment of food allergy in conjunction with restriction of main causative allergens – i.e. avoiding the known foodstuffs which cause the symptoms. FISONS

Napratec

A combination pack containing tablets of naproxen (a non-steroidal anti-inflammatory drug) and tablets of cytotec (a prostaglandin which protects the gastroduodenal mucosa against ulcer induced by NSAIDs) for the treatment of rheumatoid arthritis, osteoarthritis and ankylosing spondylitis and prevention of drug-induced gastric ulcer.

SEARLE

Naproysn

Tablets, suppositories, suspension or granules containing naproxen for the treatment of arthritis, acute gout and acute musculoskeletal disorders (such as sprains and strains, direct trauma, lumbosacral pain, tenosynovitis).

SYNTEX PHARMACEUTCIALS

Nardil

Tablets containing phenelzine a monoamine oxidase inhibitor for the symptoms of depressive illness, especially where phobic symptoms are present or where treatment with other anti-depressants has failed. PARKE DAVIS

Naseptin

Cream containing chlorhexidine hydrochloride (an antiseptic) and neomycin sulphate (an antibiotic) for bacterial infections of the nose (boils for example). ICI

Navidrex

Tablets containing cyclopenthiazide a diuretic and also used to treat mild to moderate high blood pressure. CIBA

Navispare

Tablets containing cyclopenthiazide and amiloride (diuretics) to treat high blood pressure. CIBA

Negram

Suspension or tablets containing nalidixic acid (an antibiotic) used to treat urinary tract infections.

SANOFI WINTHROP

Neocon 1/35

Combined oral contraceptive containing norethisterone and ethinyloestradiol. ORTHO

Neo-Cortef Eye/Ear Drops; Neo-Cortef Eye/ Ear Ointment

Drops and ointment containing hydrocortisone acetate (a corticosteroid) and neomycin sulphate (an antibiotic) for the short-term treatment of steroid responsive conditions of the eye when prophylactic treatment is also required, after excluding the presence of fungal and viral diseases since these organisms are not destroyed by antibiotics and their growth could be encouraged by the steroid. Blepharitis and otitis externa. CUSI (UK) LTD

Neogest

Progestogen only 'mini pill' containing levonorgestrel and norgestrel. SCHERING

Neotigason

Capsules containing acitretin used as a vitamin A derivative for the treatment of severe psoriasis. ROCHE

Neo Mercazole

Tablets containing carbimazole (an anti-thyroid agent) for conditions where reduction of thyroid functions is needed. ROCHE NICHOLAS

Neosporin Eye Drops

A topical antibacterial agent containing polymyxin b sulphate, neomycin sulphate and gramicidin for the prevention and treatment of external bacterial infections of the eye, after the removal of foreign bodies and before and after eye surgery. CUSI (UK) LTD

Nericur Gel 5/10

Gel containing benzoyl peroxide for acne. SCHERING

Nerisone Cream, Oily Cream and Ointment

Creams and ointment containing diflucortolone valerate (a corticosteroid) for dry skin conditions such as eczema where there's no infection. Stronger formulated Nerisone forte available. SCHERING

Neurontin

Capsules containing gabapentin (an anticonvulsant) to treat epilepsy. PARKE DAVIS

Nicabate

Patches containing a drug reservoir of nicotine for the relief of nicotine withdrawal symptoms associated with giving up smoking.

MARION MERRELL DOW

Nicotinell TTS
Patches containing nicotine to help give up smoking. GEIGY

Niferex Elixir
An iron supplement elixir for the prevention and treatment of uncomplicated iron-deficiency anaemia.
TILLOMED LABORATORIES LTD

Niferex-150
Capsules used as an iron supplement for the treatment of uncomplicated iron-deficiency anaemia.
TILLOMED LABORATORIES LTD

nitrazepam
A benzodiazepine used to treat insomnia.

Nitrocontin Continus Tablets
Tablets containing glyceryl trinitrate for angina. ASTA MEDICA

Nitro-Dur
Patches containing glyceryl trinitrate for the prevention of angina. SCHERING-PLOUGH

Nizoral
Anti-fungal tablets containing ketoconazole for severe fungus infections and vaginal thrush which isn't responsive to other therapy. JANSSEN

Nizoral Cream
Cream containing ketoconazole. Uses include fungal skin infections including athlete's foot.
JANSSEN

Nizoral Shampoo
Shampoo containing ketoconazole to relieve scaling and itching associated with seborrhoeic dermatitis, dandruff and pityriasis versicolor – a fungal skin condition. JANSSEN

Noctec
Capsules containing chloral hydrate for the treatment of insomnia. SQUIBB

Nobrium (Not on the NHS)
Capsules containing medazepam for the short-term treatment of anxiety.
ROCHE

Nordox
Capsules containing doxycycline (an antibiotic) for the treatment of genito-urinary tract infections, soft tissue infections and pneumonia. PANPHARMA

Norgeston
Progestogen-only mini pill containing levonorgestrel.
SCHERING

Noriday
Progestogen-only contraceptive containing norethisterone. SYNTEX

Norimin
Combined oral contraceptive containing norethisterone and ethinyloestradiol. SYNTEX

Norinyl-1
Combined oral contraceptive containing norethisterone and mestranol. SYNTEX

Normacol/Normacol Plus
Granules of a water-absorbing vegetable gum sterculia for the treatment of constipation and other conditions needing a high-fibre regime. Normacol Plus also contains frangula and is used for constipation and the initiation of bowel action after rectal surgery. NORGINE

Normison (Generic on the NHS)
Capsules containing temazepam for the short-term treatment of insomnia. WYETH

Noroxin Opthalmic Solution
Vials containing norfloxacin (a broad spectrum antibacterial agent) for superficial infections of the eye, its lids and local tissues.
MERCK SHARP & DOHME LTD

Nuelin
Tablets and liquid containing theophylline for the treatment of asthma and bronchitis.
3M HEALTH CARE

Nu-Seals Aspirin
Aspirin tablets for high and prolonged dosage of aspirin.
LILLY

Nutraplus Cream
A cream whose constituents include 10% urea which provides a moisturising effect lasting five to six hours, for the treatment of dry or damaged skin. GALDERMA (UK) LTD

Nuvelle
Hormone replacement therapy containing the oestrogen oestradiol valerate and the progestogen levonorgestrel. SCHERING

Nystan
Suspension and tablets containing nystatin (an antifungal antibiotic). Uses include oral thrush and intestinal thrush. SQUIBB

Nytol
Tablets containing diphenhydramine hydrochloride used as an aid to the relief of temporary sleep disturbance.
STAFFORD-MILLER

Oestradiol Implants
HRT implants containing oestradiol for post-menopausal symptoms due to oestrogen deficiency.
ORGANON

Olbetam
Capsules containing acipimox for the treatment of high cholesterol.
FARMITALIA CARLO ERBA

Opticrom Aqueous Eye Drops, Eye Ointment
Drops or ointment containing sodium cromoglycate for the relief and treatment of allergic eye disease including hay fever and allergic conjuncitivits. FISONS

Orelox Tablets
Tablets containing cefpodoxime proxetil a bactericidal cephalosporin antibiotic active against a wide range of organisms. Used in the treatment of upper and lower respiratory tract infections. ROUSSEL

Orlept
Tablets containing sodium valproate for the treatment of epilepsy. CP PHARMACEUTICALS

Ortho-Dienoestrol Cream
Cream containing dienoestrol for intravaginal use in the treatment of atrophic vaginitis and kraurosis vulvae in postmenopausal women.
ORTHO

Ortho-Gynest Cream and Pessaries
Cream and pessaries containing oestriol, a naturally occurring oestrogen, for the treatment of atrophic vaginitis and kraurosis vulvae – a degenerative, dry condition – in post menopausal women.
ORTHO

Orthonovin 1/50
Combined oral contraceptive containing norethisterone and mestranol – also used for disorders such as heavy, irregular or painful periods.
ORTHO

Orudis
Capsules containing ketoprofen for the management of rheumatoid arthritis, osteoarthritis, ankylosing spondylitis, and disorders such as bursitis, capsulitis, tendonitis, fibrositis, back pain, painful musculo-skeletal conditions, painful periods, acute gout and control of pain and inflammation following orthopaedic surgery. Suppositories are not recommended for painful periods. RHONE-POULENC RORER

Oruvail Gel
Gel containing ketoprofen for the relief of painful musculoskeletal conditions such as sports injuries, sprains, strains and contusions. RHONE-POULENC RORER

Ossopan
Tablets or granules containing calcium and phosphorous for osteoporosis, rickets and osteomalacia and during lactation. SANOFI WINTHROP

Otomize Ear Spray
Spray containing dexamethasone (a corticosteroid) and neomycin sulphate (an antibiotic) for the treatment of otitis externa. STAFFORD-MILLER

Otosporin
Ear drops containing polymyxin b sulphate, neomycin sulphate and hydrocortisone for otitis externa with bacterial infection. WELLCOME

Ovran/Ovran 30/ Ovranette
Combined oestrogen progestogen contraceptive pills containing levonorgestrel and ethinyloestradiol. WYETH

Ovysmen
Combined oral contraceptive containing norethisterone and ethinyloestradiol. ORTHO

Oxazepam Tablets
Tablets containing oxazepam (a benzodiazepine) for short-term treatment of anxiety including insomnia associated with anxiety. WYETH

Oxivent
Metered inhaler containing oxitropium bromide (an anticholinergic bronchodilator). Uses include the management of airways obstruction in patients suffering from stable chronic asthma. BOEHRINGER INGELHEIM

Oxypertine
Capsules containing the antipsychotic drug oxypertine. Uses include the short term treatment of severe anxiety. SANOFI WINTHROP

Palaprin Forte
Tablets containing aloxiprin, an analgesic/anti-inflammatory agent used in rheumatoid arthritis, oestoarthritis and other 'rheumatic' conditions where high dosage salicylate therapy is indicated. ROCHE NICHOLAS

Paludrine Tablets
Tablets containing proguanil hydrochloride, an effective antimalarial agent for the prevention and suppression of malaria. ICI

Panadol and Panadol Extra
Tablets, capsules, soluble and junior sachets, baby and infant suspension containing paracetamol for the treatment of most painful and feverish conditions for example, headache including migraine, toothache, sore throat, colds, influenza, rheumatic pain and period pain. Panadol Extra available as tablets and also contain the stimulant caffeine.
STERLING HEALTH

paracetamol
A non-narcotic analgesic to treat mild to moderate pain.

Paramax
Tablets or powder containing paracetamol and metoclopramide hydrochloride for the symptomatic relief of migraine. BENCARD

Parlodel
Tablets or capsules containing bromocriptine mesylate (a dopamine agonist). Uses include the treatment of Parkinson's disease. SANDOZ

Pavacol-D
Cough mixture containing pholcodine (a cough-suppressant) for the symptomatic treatment of dry troublesome coughs.
BOEHRINGER INGELHEIM

Pendramine
Tablets containing D-penicillamine. Uses include the treatment of severe active rheumatoid arthritis. ASTA MEDICA

Pentasa Slow Release Tablets and Pentasa Mesalazine Enema
Tablets or enema containing mesalazine. Tablets used for the maintenance of remission in mild to moderate ulcerative colitis and enema for the treatment of ulcerative colitis affecting the distal colon and rectum. BROCADES.

pentazocine
A narcotic analgesic to treat moderate to severe pain.

Pepcid
Tablets containing famotidine used for the treatment of ulcers and in the treatment of gastro-oesophageal disease.
THOMAS MORSON PHARMACEUTICALS

Periactin
Tablets containing cyproheptadine hydrochloride. Periactin is a

serotonin and histamine antagonist with anticholinergic and sedative properties. Its beneficial action affects the local tissues, central nervous system and peripheral nerves, as well as the brain. Uses include the treatment of itchy skin conditions such as dermatitis and eczema; allergic reactions to insect bites, hay fever, perennial rhinitis, allergic conjunctivitis, urticaria, and the itching of chickenpox; migraine and as an appetitite stimulant. MERCK SHARP & DOHME

Pertofran
Tablets containing desipramine hydrochloride for the symptoms of depression. GEIGY

Phenergan
Tablets containing promethazine hydrochloride, elixir, or injection. Uses include allergic conditions, insomnia, as an anti-emetic and as a sedative in children. RHONE-POULENC RORER

pholcodine linctus
A cough suppressant.

Pholcomed D Linctus, Pholcomed Diabetic Forte Linctus (Not on the NHS)
Linctus containing pholcodine for the relief of irritating, unproductive coughs. MEDO PHARMACEUTICALS

Phyllocontin
Tablets containing aminophylline hydrate (a bronchodilator) for the treatment and prevention of bronchospasm associated with asthma and chronic bronchitis. NAPP

Piriton
A potent antihistamine – chlorpheniramine maleate – for the control of allergic conditions. ALLEN & HANBURYS

Plaquenil
Tablets containing hydroxychloroquine sulphate – uses include rheumatoid arthritis. SANOFI WINTHROP

Plendil
Tablets containing felodipine for the management of high blood pressure. SCHWARZ PHARMA

Polyfax Ointment
Anitbacterial ointment containing polymyxin b sulphate and zinc bacitracin for the treatment of infected wounds, burns, impetigo for example and and secondarily infected skin lesions of scabies, pediculosis – an infestation with lice – athlete's foot and dermatitis. CUSI (UK) LTD

Polyfax Opthalmic Ointment
Antibacterial ointment containing polymyxin b sulphate and bacitracin zinc for the treatment of bacterial infections of the eye and its surrounding tissues including conjunctivits and ulcerative blepharitis. CUSI (UK) LTD

Polytrim Eye Drops
Antibacterial eye drops containing trimethoprim and polymyxin b sulphate for the treatment and prevention of external bacterial eye infections including conjunctivitis and ulcerative blepharitis, also as a preventive measure after the removal of foreign bodies and before and after eye surgery. CUSI (UK) LTD

Polytrim Opthalmic Ointment
An antibacterial ointment containing trimethoprim and polymyxin b sulphate for the treatment and prevention of external bacterial eye infections and surrounding tissues including conjunctivitis, ulcerative blepharitis with associated conjunctivitis. CUSI (UK) LTD

Ponstan
Capsules or paediatric suspension containing mefenamic acid. Uses include arthritis, painful periods and menorrhagia. PARKE-DAVIS RESEARCH

Posafilin
Acidic ointment containing podophyllum resin and salicylic acid for the treatment of plantar warts. NORGINE

Pragmatar Cream
Cream containing coal tar, sulphur and salicylic acid for the treatment of dandruff,other seborrhoeic conditions, and common scaly skin disorders. BIOGLAN

Precortisyl
Tablets containing prednisolone (used as a corticosteroid) to treat Crohn's disease, ulcerative colitis, allergies and other disorders including blood disorders, renal disorders and rheumatic conditions. ROUSSEL

Predenema
Enema containing prednisolone for the local treatment of ulcerative colitis. PHARMAX

Prednesol Tablets
Tablets containing prednisolone sodium phosphate(a steroid). Many diseases may be improved by the careful use of strong medicines like this, which

mainly work by reducing inflammation in the body. Uses include bronchial asthma, rheumatoid arthritis, ulcerative colitis, Crohn's disease. GLAXO

Preferid Cream/Ointment
Cream containing budesonide (a corticosteroid) for the treatment of eczema, dermatitis and psoriasis (except widespread plaque psoriasis). BROCADES

Pregaday
Tablets containing ferrous fumarate and anhydrous folic acid for prevention of iron deficiency and megaloblastic anaemia of pregnancy. EVANS

Premarin Tablets
Tablets containing naturally conjugated oestrogens for menopausal and postmenopausal oestrogen therapy in women without a uterus. WYETH

Prempak-C
Tablets containing naturally conjugated oestrogens and also tablets containing norgestrel – menopausal and postmenopausal oestrogen therapy. WYETH

Prepulsid
Tablets or suspension containing cisapride monohydrate a gastrointestinal prokinetic agent i.e. it increases the speed of downward propulsion of digesting food. Uses include gastro-oesophagul reflux and dyspepsia. JANSSEN

Prescal
Tablets containing isradipine used to reduce high blood pressure. CIBA

Primalan
Antihistamine tablets containing mequitazine for allergic conditions such as hay fever, perennial rhinitis, urticaria, or allergic reactions associated with bites and stings. RHONE-POULENC RORER

Primolut N
Hormonal preparation containing the progestogen norethisterone for the treatment of premenstrual syndrome, postponement of menstruation, endometriosis and menorrhagia – heavy or prolonged periods. SCHERING

Prioderm
Lotion for the treatment of head and pubic lice infestations and scabies, containing malathion. Cream shampoo suitable for the treatment of head and pubic lice. NAPP

Pripsen
Powder containing piperazine phosphate and sennosides, the main active ingredient of the laxative senna fruit, to treat threadworm and roundworm. Pripsen acts by paralysing the adult worms which are then expelled by the gentle laxative action of standardised senna. RECKITT & COLMAN

Pro-Actidil
Tablets containing triprolidine hydrochloride (an antihistamine) for hay fever and allergic skin conditions. WELLCOME

Proctofoam HC
Foam containing hydrocortisone acetate and pramoxine hydrochloride for the short-term (not more than five to seven days) relief of the symptoms of itching, irritation, discomfort or pain associated with noninfective anal or perianal conditions. STAFFORD-MILLER

Proctosedyl
Suppositories or ointment containing cinchocaine hydrochloride (a local anaesthetic) and hydrocortisone (a corticosteroid) to soothe itching and relieve inflammation in piles and anal itching. ROUSSEL

Proflex
Cream containing ibuprofen for relief of rheumatic and muscular pain, backache, sprains and strains. ZYMA

Progesic
Tablets containing fenoprofen for the treatment of arthritis and for the relief of mild to moderate pain and fever. LILLY

Progynova
HRT tablets containing oestradiol valerate – an oestrogen preparation for the short-term treatment of climacteric symptoms in postmenopausal women. SCHERING

Prominal
Tablets containing methylphenobarbitone for the treatment of epilepsy. SANOFI WINTHROP

Propaderm Cream/ Ointment
Cream or ointment containing beclomethasone dipropionate (a topical steroid) a strong and rapidly effective treatment for inflamed skin conditions such as eczema, dermatitis and psoriasis. GLAXO

Pro-vent
Capsules containing theophylline for the prevention and treatment of bronchial smooth-muscle constriction in asthma and chronic bronchitis. WELLCOME

Provera
Tablets containing medroxyprogesterone acetate (a progestogen). Uses include the treatment of mild to moderate endometriosis. UPJOHN LTD

Psoradrate Cream
Cream containing dithranol used to treat psoriasis. PROCTER & GAMBLE

Psorigel
An emollient coal tar gel for use on the skin and the scalp for the relief and treatment of inflammation and itching in eczema, psoriasis and dermatitis, for example. GALDERMA (UK) LTD

Pulmadil
Inhaler providing rimiterol hydrobromide (a bronchodilator) for asthma and bronchitis. 3M HEALTH CARE

Pulmicort Inhaler, Pulmicort Respules (suspension for nebulisation), Pulmicort Turbohaler (powder inhaler)
Pulmicort range contains budesonide, a corticosteroid. Inhaled budesonide possesses a local anti-inflammatory action in the lungs without giving rise to systemic corticosteroid effects. Pulmicort is recommended in patients with bronchial asthma. ASTRA

Pyralvex
Analgesic anti-inflammatory with an antiseptic base to treat the pain of mouth ulcers and denture irritation. Contains salicylic acid and rhubarb extract. NORGINE

Pyrogastrone
Tablets containing carbenoxolone sodium, dried aluminium hydroxide, magnesium trisilicate in a base containing sodium bicarbonate and alginic acid for the treatment of oesophegeal inflammation, erosions and ulcers due to hiatus hernia or other conditions causing gastro-oesophageal reflux and for the relief of heartburn, flatulence and other symptoms associated with

reflux oesophagitis. Also available as liquid.

SANOFI WINTHROP

Quellada

Lotion containing gamma benzene hexachloride for the treatment of scabies.

STAFFORD-MILLER

Questran, Questran A

Powder containing anhydrous cholestyramine for high cholesterol. BRISTOL-MYERS

Quinocort Cream

Cream containing potassium hydroxyquinoline sulphate and hydrocortisone for the treatment of infected eczema, intertrigo and other skin conditions. QUINODERM

Quinoderm Cream Hydrocortisone 1%

Cream containing benzoyl peroxide (a keratolytic), potassium hydroxyquinoline sulphate (an antifungal agent) and hydrocortisone (a corticosteroid with anti-inflammatory properties) for the treatment of acne, acneform eruptions and folliculitis especially where inflamed lesions are present.

QUINODERM

Rastinon Tablets

Tablets containing tolbutamide an anti-diabetic drug. HOECHST

Rehidrat Blackcurrant/ Lemon and Lime/Orange

Blackcurrant or orange flavoured oral sugar/ electrolyte powder for use in the treatment of diarrhoea.

SEARLE

Relifex

Tablets and suspension containing nabumetone a non-acidic non-steroidal anti-inflammatory agent which, inhibits the production of prostaglandin which is the cause of many of the symptoms of the arthritis. Used for the treatment of osteoarthritis and rheumatoid arthritis. BENCARD

Remedeine

Analgesic containing paracetamol and dihydrocodeine for severe pain including severe acute back pain, sports injuries and fractures. NAPP

Revanil

Tablets containing lisuride maleate for the treatment of Parkinson's disease. ROCHE

Rheumox 600/Capsules
Tablets or capsules containing azapropazone dihydrate (a non-steroidal anti-inflammatory drug). Uses include the treatment of arthritis and prevention of gout. WYETH

Rhinocort and Rhinocort Aqua
Aerosol and pump spray containing corticosteroid budesonide for seasonal and perennial, allergic rhinitis and vasomotor rhinitis. ASTRA

Rhinolast Nasal Spray
Antihistamine spray containing azelastine hydrochloride for the treatment of perennial and seasonal allergic rhinitis including hay fever. ASTA MEDICA

Ridaura
Tablets containing auranofin, an orally active gold preparation for rheumatoid arthritis. BENCARD

Rifadin
Antibiotic capsules or syrup containing rifampicin. Uses include tuberculosis and prevention of meningococcal meningitis. MARION MERRELL DOW

Rifater
Antibiotic combination tablets containing isoniazid, pyrazinamide and rifampicin for the treatment of pulmonary tuberculosis. MARION MERRELL DOW

Rifinah
Antibiotic combination tablets containing rifampicin and isoniazid for the treament of tuberculosis. MARION MERRELL DOW

Rimactane/Rimactane Syrup
Capsules and syrup containing rifampicin (an antibiotic) used to treat infections such as tuberculosis. It's also used to help prevent the spread of some forms of meningitis. CIBA

Rimactazid Combined Tablets
Tablets containing rifampicin and isoniazid used to treat tuberculosis. CIBA

Rinatec
Metered dose inhaler containing ipratropium bromide (an antcholinergic drug which acts as an antagonist against the muscarinic receptors of the mucoserous glands, and so prevents some of their overstimulation). For the treatment and management of watery rhinorrhoea

associated with perennial rhinitis. BOEHRINGER INGELHEIM

Rivotril
Tablets, or ampoules for injection, containing clonazepam for epilepsy.
ROCHE

Rhinolast Nasal Spray
Nasal spray containing azelastine hydrochloride (an anti-allergic agent) for use in the treatment of perennial and seasonal allergic rhinitis, including hay fever. ASTA MEDICA

Roaccutane
Capsules containing isotretinoin for the treatment of acne. ROCHE

Robaxin 750
Tablets containing methocarbamol used as a short-term adjunct to the symptomatic treatment of acute musculo-skeletal disorders associated with painful muscle spasms. WYETH

Robaxisal Forte (Not on the NHS)
Tablet containing methocarbamol and acetylsalicylic acid used in the short-term management of pain and skeletal muscle spasm associated with musculo-skeletal disorders such as lumbago, fibrositis, sprains, strains etc. WYETH

Rohypnol (Not on the NHS)
Tablets containing flunitrazepam (a benzodiazepine compound) for the short-term treatment of insomnia when it's severe.
ROCHE

Rynacrom 4% Nasal Spray/Cartridges/ Nasal Drops
Sodium cromoglycate for the preventive treatment of allergic rhinitis (hayfever and perennial). FISONS

Rynacrom Compound
A metered dose of sodium cromoglycate and xylometazoline hydrochloride (a decongestant) for the prevention, relief and treatment of allergic rhinitis (such as hayfever and perennial rhinitis) where this is accompanied by nasal congestion. FISONS

Sabril Tablets and Sachets
Tablets and sachets containing vigabatrin recommended as 'add-on' treatment of epilepsy which is not satisfactorily controlled by other anti-epileptic drugs.
MARION MERRELL DOW

Salazopyrin
Tablets containing sulphasalazine. Uses include

the treatment of rheumatoid arthritis and Crohn's disease and for the induction and maintenance of ulcerative colitis remission. KABI PHARMACIA

Salbulin
Inhaler providing salbutamol for asthma and bronchitis.
3M HEALTH CARE

Saluric
Tablets containing chlorothiazide (a diuretic and antihypertensive agent) for fluid retention and high blood pressure. MERCK SHARP & DOHME LTD

Sandocal 1000
Tablets containing calcium lactate gluconate and calcium carbonate. This medicine is taken to slow down or stop calcium loss from bones in osteoporosis. It is also taken to treat calcium deficiency.
SANDOZ

Sanomigran
Tablets containing an antihistamine pizotifen used to prevent migraine headaches. SANDOZ

Scheriproct Ointment and Suppositories
A corticosteroid with anaesthetic and antihistamine properties containing prednisolone hexanoate and dibucaine hydrochloride for the symptomatic relief of haemorrhoids and anal and vulva itching in the short-term (five to seven days).
SCHERING

Schering PC4
Oral contraceptive used as an emergency after sexual intercourse has taken place – the morning-after pill – combines oestrogen and progestogen – ethinyloestradiol and levonorgestrel. SCHERING

Scopoderm TTS
Patches containing hyoscine (an anti-emetic) used to prevent the symptoms of travel sickness. CIBA

Secadrex
Tablets containing acebutolol (a beta-blocker) and hydrochlorothiazide (a diuretic) for mild to moderate high blood pressure. Secadrex has been shown to be particulary suitable for elderly patients.
RHONE-POULENC RORER

Sectral
Capsules containing acebutolol (a beta-blocker) for high blood pressure, angina and abnormal heart rhythms.
RHONE-POULENC RORER.

Semprex
Capsules containing the antihistamine acrivastine for the treatment of hay fever and urticaria. WELLCOME

senna
A stimulant laxative for constipation.

Senokot (Generic on the NHS)
Tablets, granules or syrup containing senna for the management of constipation. RECKITT & COLMAN

Septrin
Antibiotic tablets and suspension containing trimethoprim and sulphamethoxazole. Uses include infections of the respiratory tract, genito-urinary tract, gastro-intestinal tract, and skin infections. WELLCOME

Serc/Serc-16
Tablets containing betahistine dihydrochloride (a histamine analogue – chemically similar in structure and action to naturally occurring histamine) for vertigo, tinnitus and hearing loss associated with Menière's syndrome. DUPHAR

Serevent
Inhaler and diskhaler containing salmeterol and lactose for asthma. ALLEN & HANBURYS

Seroxat
Tablets containing paroxetine hydrochloride used for the treatment of symptoms of depressive illness of all types including depression accompanied by anxiety. SMITHKLINE BEECHAM PHARMACEUTICALS

simple linctus
Linctus containing glycerol to sooth an irritating cough.

Sinthrome
Tablets containing nicoumalone (an anticoagulant) for the treatment and prevention of thromboembolic diseases. GEIGY

Siopel
Barrier cream containing the antiseptic cetrimide and water-repellant dimethicone uses include nappy rash. ICI

Skinoren
Cream containing azelaic acid for the treatment of acne. SCHERING

Slow-Fe
Tablets containing dried ferrous sulphate for the

treatment and prevention of iron deficiency anaemia. CIBA

Slow-Fe Folic
Tablets containing dried ferrous sulphate and folic acid for iron and folic acid deficiency in pregnancy. CIBA

Slow-Trasicor
Tablets containing oxprenolol hydrochloride (a beta-blocker) for high blood pressure and angina. CIBA

Sno Phenicol
Drops containing chloramphenicol (an antibiotic) for the treatment of bacterial eye infections.
SMITH & NEPHEW

sodium picosulphate
A stimulant laxative used for constipation.

Sofradex Ear/Eye Drops and Ointment
Corticosteroid antibiotic drops and ointment containing framycetin sulphate, gramicidin and dexamethasone for otitis externa, blepharitis and the short-term treatment of steroid responsive conditions of the eye when prophylactic antibiotic treatment is required, after excluding the presence of fungal and viral disease since these are not destroyed by the antibiotics and the steroids may encourage their growth.
ROUSSEL

Soframycin Skin Ointment
Antibiotic skin ointment containing framycetin sulphate and gramicidin for primary infections such as infective dermatitis, folliculitis, impetigo and boils, and secondary infections in cuts, scratches, burns, eczema etc. ROUSSEL

Soframycin Sterile Eye Drops/Ointment
Antibiotic ointment and drops containing framycetin sulphate. Uses include the treatment of bacterial infections of the eye, notably conjunctivitis and blepharitis, for styes, corneal abrasions and burns and to prevent infection after the removal of foreign bodies. ROUSSEL

Sofra-tulle
A sterile lano-paraffin gauze dressing impregnated with framycetin sulphate. It has a wide range of antibacterial activity and is an ideal dressing for immediate use in a variety of infected lesions e.g. burns and bites; and secondary infected skin

conditions such as eczema and dermatitis. ROUSSEL

Solpadeine
Soluble tablets containing paracetamol, codeine phosphate and caffeine for the treatment of mild to moderate pain. Suitable for migraine, headache, rheumatic pain, period pain, toothache, neuralgia, sore throat and feverishness and symptomatic treatment of colds and flu. STERLING HEALTH

Solpadol
Soluble tablets containing combined analgesics – paracetamol and codeine phosphate for the relief of severe pain. SANOFI WINTHROP

Somnite
A suspension containing nitrazepam (a benzodiazepine) for the short-term treatment of insomnia where daytime sedation is acceptable. NORGINE

Soneryl
Tablets containing butobarbitone (a barbiturate) used for severe, intractable insomnia. RHONE-POULENC RORER

Sorbitrate
Tablets containing isosorbide dinitrate (a vasodilator) which can help to prevent an attack of chest pain (angina).
STUART PHARMACEUTICALS

Sorbichew
Tablets containing isosorbide dinitrate (a vasodilator) to help prevent an attack of chest pain (angina).
STUART PHARMACEUTICALS

Sorbid SA
Sustained release capsules containing isosorbide dinitrate (a vasodilator) to help prevent an attack of chest pain (angina).
STUART PHARMACEUTICALS

Spasmonal
Capsules containing alverine citrate (an antispasmodic) for the relief of smooth muscle spasm in conditions such as irritable bowel disease and painful periods. NORGINE

Sporanox
Capsules containing itraconazole for the treatment of oral and vaginal thrush and fungal skin infections including athlete's foot.
JANSSEN

Stafoxil Capsules
Capsules containing flucloxacillin (an antibiotic) for the treatment of infections such as respiratory tract infections, infections of the

skin and soft tissues and generalised infections.

BROCADES

Stemetil

Tablets, injection, suppositories, or syrup containing prochlorperazine maleate (a phenothiazine neuroleptic – a medicine that is also used to treat mental illness). Uses include vertigo due to Meniere's syndrome, labyrinthitis, and for nausea and vomiting from whatever cause including that associated with migraine; and as an adjunct to the short-term management of anxiety. Effervescent sachets available.

RHONE-POULENC RORER

Sudafed Tablets and Elixir, Sudafed SA

Tablets or elixir containing pseudoephedrine hydrochloride (a decongestant) for relief of allergic rhinitis, vasomotor rhinitis, the common cold and influenza. WELLCOME

Sudocrem

Antiseptic healing cream containing benzoyl alcohol and benzyl benzoate for nappy rash, eczema, minor burns etc. TOSARA

Surgam

Capsules and tablets containing tiaprofenic acid a non-steroidal anti-inflammatory agent with marked analgesic properties. Uses include arthritis, low back pain, musculo-skeletal disorders such as fibrositis, capsulitis, sprains and strains.

ROUSSEL

Surmontil

Tablets containing trimipramine (an antidepressant) used for the treatment of depression especially where sleep disturbance, anxiety or agitation is a problem.

RHONE-POULENC RORER

Symmetrel Capsules

Capsules containing amantadine hydrochloride used to treat Parkinson's disease and as an anti-viral drug. GEIGY

Symmetrel Syrup

Syrup containing amantadine hydrochloride for Parkinson's disease and herpes zoster (shingles). GEIGY

Synalar Cream/Ointment

Cream or ointment containing fluocinolone acetonide, a topical corticosteroid for a wide range of skin conditions such as eczema dermatitis and psoriasis. Also available as Synalar Cream 1 in 4 Dilution and Synalar Ointment 1 in 4 Dilution and Synalar Cream 1 in 10 dilution. ICI

Synalar Gel
Gel containing fluocinolone acetonide, a topical corticosteroid designed for application to the scalp and other hairy regions as well as elsewhere on the body. Specifically useful for seborrhoea, seborrhoeic dermatitis and psoriasis of the scalp. ICI

Synalar C Cream and Ointment
Cream and ointment containing the steroid fluocinolone acetidone and clioquinol (an antibacterial and antifungal agent) for inflammatory skin conditions, including eczema, dermatitis, seborrhoea and intertrigo, where secondary bacterial and/or fungal infection is present or likely to occur. ICI

Synalar N Cream and Ointment
Cream and ointment containing the steroid fluocinolone acetonide and antibacterial agent neomycin sulphate for inflammatory skin conditions, including eczema, dermatitis, seborrhoea and intertrigo, where secondary bacterial infection is present or is likely to occur. ICI

Synphase
Oral contraceptive containing norethisterone and ethinyloestradiol. SYNTEX

Tagamet
Tablets, syrup, injection and infusion containing cimetidine which inhibits gastric secretion and reduces pepsin output and is used for the treatment of peptic ulcers and other conditions where reduction of gastric acid has been shown to be beneficial, such as reflux oesophagitis.
SMITH KLINE & FRENCH

Tarcortin
Cream containing hydrocortisone and coal tar for eczema and psoriasis.
STAFFORD-MILLER

Tarivid
Tablets and infusion containing ofloxacin – an antibacterial agent used in the treatment of upper and lower urinary tract infections, lower respiratory tract infections, and gonorrhoea, for example.
ROUSSEL/HOECHST

Tegretol/Tegretol Retard
Tablets, chewtabs, or liquid containing carbamazepine for epilepsy. Retard available as divitabs – tablets able to be taken whole or in half. Tegretol Retard is also used to treat a painful condition of the face called trigeminal neuralgia. GEIGY

Temazepam Capsules/ Tablets
Capsules or tablets containing temazepam (a benzodiazepine). Uses include the short-term treatment of insomnia and for premedication before minor surgery.

Tenif
Capsules containing atenolol (a beta-blocker) and nifedipine (a calcium blokcer) for management of high blood pressure and angina.
STUART PHARMACEUTICALS

Tenoret 50
Tablets containing atenolol (a beta-blocker) and chlorthalidone (a diuretic) for the mangement of high blood pressure. A combination of low effective doses making this particularly suited to the older patient.
STUART PHARMACEUTICALS

Tenoretic
Tablets containing a combination of two drugs, atenolol (a beta-blocker) and chlorthalidone (a diuretic) used to treat high blood pressure. STUART PHARMACEUTICAL

Tenormin
Tablets containing atenolol (a beta-blocker) used to treat high blood pressure or chest pain (angina).
STUART PHARMACEUTICAL

Tetmosol Soap
Soap containing monosulfiram (a parasiticide) for the treatment and prevention of scabies. ICI

Tetmosol Solution
Liquid containing monosulfiram (a parasiticide) for the treatment and prevention of scabies. ICI

Theo-Dur
Tablets containing theophyline, a bronchodilator used in the symptomatic or preventive treatment of bronchospasm associated with chronic obstructive airways disease including asthma and bronchitis. ASTRA

Thephorin
Tablets containing phenindamine tartrate, an antihistamine used to give

symptomatic relief in allergic disorders such as hay fever, allergic rhinitis, urticaria, insect bites and stings.

SINCLAIR PHARMACEUTICALS

Tigason
Capsules containing etretinate used as a vitamin A derivative to treat severe psoriasis. ROCHE

Tilade
Tilade Mint Inhaler and Tilade Mint Syncroner containing nedocromil sodium for the treatment of bronchial asthma and other reversible obstructive airways diseases. FISONS

Tildiem
Tablets containing diltiazem hydrochloride (a calcium antagonist) for the treatment of angina. Tildiem Retard Tablets also for high blood pressure. LOREX

Tildiem LA
Capsules containing diltiazem hydrochloride (a calcium antagonist) for mild to moderate high blood pressure. LOREX

Timodine
A corticosteroid cream containing hydrocortisone, nystatin (an antifungal agent) and antiseptic benzalkonium chloride for the treatment of skin conditions including intertrigo, seborrhoeic dermatitis, pruritis ani and vulvae and nappy rash where thrush is a factor.

RECKITT & COLMAN

Tinaderm M Cream
Cream containing tolnaftate (an anti-fungal agent) and nystatin (an antibiotic) for the treatment of fungal nail and skin infections including athlete's foot, intertrigo, nappy rash. SCHERING-PLOUGH

Tineafax Cream, Powder
Cream containing tolnaftate for the treatment of athlete's foot and ringworm. Powder for the prevention of athlete's foot. WELLCOME

Tinset
Tablets containing oxatomide for the symptomatic control of allergic rhinitis, conjunctivitis and urticaria and other conditions responsive to drugs with anti-histaminic properties. Food allergy.

JANSSEN

Tofranil/Tofranil Syrup
Tablets containing imipramine used to treat depression. Can also be used to treat bed-wetting in children. GEIGY

Topal
Tablets containing dried aluminium hydroxide gel, light magnesium carbonate, alginic acid for the relief of discomfort due to gastric reflux in conditions such as heartburn, reflux oesophagitis, hiatus hernia, gastritis, acid dyspepsia.
PIERRE FABRE LTD

Topicycline
Antibiotic solution containing tetracycline hydochloride for the treatment of acne.
PROCTER & GAMBLE

Topilar Cream and Ointment
Cream and ointment containing fluclorolone acetonide (a topical corticosteroid) for the treatment of eczema and dermatitis. BIOGLAN

Totamol
Tablets containing atenolol. Uses include the management of high blood pressure and angina. CP PHARMACEUTICALS

Trancopal
Tablets containing chlormezanone uses include the short-term treatment of anxiety, insomnia and as an adjunct to the treatment of acute musculoskeletal disorders associated with painful muscle spasm.
SANOFI WINTHROP

Tranxene (Not on the NHS)
Capsules containing dipotassium clorazepate (a benzodiazepine) for the short-term relief of anxiety.
BOEHRINGER INGELHEIM

Transiderm-Nitro
Patches containing glyceryl trinitrate to help relieve the symptoms of angina. CIBA

Trasicor
Tablets containing oxprenolol hydrochloride (a beta-blocker) for high blood pressure and angina as well as abnormal heart rhythm.
CIBA

Trasidrex
Tablets containing oxprenolol hydrochloride (a beta-blocker) and cyclopenththiazide (a diuretic) for high blood pressure. CIBA

Travogyn
Vaginal tablets or cream containing isoconazole nitrate (an anti-fungal agent) for vaginal, vulval or perineal infections such as thrush.
SCHERING

Tremonil
Tablets containing methixene hydrochloride which acts upon the body's parasympathetic (automatic) nervous system. Uses include Parkinson's disease. SANDOZ

Triadene
Combined oestrogen-progestogen oral contraceptive containing ethinyloestradiol and gestodene. SCHERING HEALTH CARE

Tri-Adocortyl Cream, Ointment and Otic Ointment
Preparations containing triamcinolone acetonide, neomycin, gramicidin, nystatin for the topical treatment of superficial bacterial infections including eczema and otitis externa. SQUIBB

Tri-Cicatrin Ointment
Ointment containing neomycin sulphate, bacitracin zinc, nystatin and hydrocortisone for dry skin conditions in which bacterial or candidal infection is present or is likely to occur. WELLCOME

Trifyba
Powder containing fibrous extract of wheat grain used in disorders of the bowel where a high fibre intake is needed. SANOFI WINTHROP

Triludan Tablets, Forte Tablets, Suspension
Tablets or suspension containing terfenadine an antihistamine for the symptomatic relief of hay fever, allergic rhinitis and allergic skin conditions. MARION MERRELL DOW

Tri-Minulet
Combined oestrogen-progestogen oral contraceptive containing ethinyloestradiol and gestodene. WYETH

Trinordial
Combined oestrogen progestogen oral contraceptive containing levonorgestrol and ethinyloestradiol. WYETH

Trinovum and Trinovum ED
Oral contraceptive containing norethisterone and ethinyloestradiol. ORTHO

Trisequens and Trisequens Forte
HRT tablets containing oestradiol and oestriol as well as oestradiol, oestriol and norethisterone acetate. NOVO NORDISK

Triptafen
Tablets containing amitriptyline hydrochloride and perphenazine for the treatment of mild to moderate depression associated with anxiety. ALLEN & HANBURYS

Trisilate
Tablets containing magnesium trisalicylate for the relief of the signs and symptoms of arthritis. NAPP

Tritace
An ACE inhibitor to treat high blood pressure containing ramipril. HOECHST

Trosyl Nail Solution
Solution containing tioconazole (a broad spectrum antifungal agent) for the topical treatment of nail infections due to susceptible fungi. PFIZER LTD

Tryptizol
Slow-release capsules and injection containing amitriptyline hydrochloride, and syrup containing amitriptyline embonate, used in the treatment of depression (especially where sedation is required).
THOMAS MORSON PHARMACEUTICALS

Tylex
Capsules containing paracetamol and codeine phosphate for the relief of severe pain. CILAG

Tyrozets
Lozenges containing tyrothricin (an antibiotic) and benzocaine (a local anaesthetic) for sore throats.
MERCK SHARP & DOHME LTD

Ultraproct Ointment/ Suppositories
Corticosteroid preparations containing fluocortolone pivalate, fluocortolone hexanoate and dibucaine hydrochloride with local anaesthetic and antihistamine properties for the symptomatic relief of haemorrhoids and of anal and vulval itching in the short-term (five to seven days).
SCHERING

Ultradil Ointment Plain and Cream Plain
A corticosteroid preparation containing fluocortolone pivalate and fluocortolone hexanoate for skin conditions such as eczema, dermatitis and psoriasis. The more highly concentrated Ultralanum Ointment Plain and Cream Plain available.
SCHERING

Unguentum Merck
An emulsion with a uniform distribution of fat and water

and emollient properties for the symptoms of dermatitis, eczema, nappy rash, ichythyosis (very dry skin), protection of raw and abraded skin areas, pruritis and related conditions where dry scaly skin is a problem, and as a pre-bathing emollient. It can also be used as a medium for various topical corticosteroids when a lower strength is needed. MERCK

Uniphyllin
Tablets containing theophylline (a bronchodilator) for the treatment and prevention of bronchospasm in asthma and chronic bronchitis. NAPP

Univer
Capsules containing verapamil hydrochloride (a calcium antagonist) for the long term treatment of mild to moderate high blood pressure and angina. RHONE-POULENC RORER

Utinor
Tablets containing norfloxacin a broad spectrum bactericidal agent for the treatment of urinary tract infections. MERCK SHARP & DOHME LTD

Vallergan
Tablets, syrup, forte syrup, containing trimeprazine tartrate (which has sedative, antihistamine and anti-emetic effects). Uses include urticaria and pruritis. RHONE-POULENC RORER

Valium Roche (Generic on the NHS)
Tablets or syrup (or ampoules for injection) containing diazepam. Uses include the short-term treatment of anxiety and muscle spasm. ROCHE

Valoid Tablets
Tablets containing cyclizine hydrochloride for the prevention and treatment of nausea and vomiting, including motion sickness and that associated with Menière's disease. WELLCOME

Vascardin
Tablets containing diluted isosorbide dinitrate (a vasodilator) uses include angina. ROCHE NICHOLAS

Ventide
Inhaler and rotacaps providing salbutamol for obstructive airways disease. ALLEN & HANBURYS

Ventolin
Inhaler, diskhaler, tablets and syrup providing salbutamol for prevention and treatment of asthma and bronchitis. ALLEN & HANBURYS

Vermox
Tablets or suspension containing mebendazole (an anthelmintic) for the treatment of worms. JANSSEN

Verrugon
Ointment containing salicylic acid for the treatment of verrucas. PICKLES

Vibrocil
Nasal spray and drops containing dimethindene maleate, phenylephrine and neomycin sulphate (a preparation with decongestant, antihistaminic and antibiotic properties) for use in common colds and rhinitis where these conditions are complicated by staphylococcal infections. ZYMA

Virudox
An anti-viral solution containing idoxuridine in dimethyl sulphoxide for the treatment of herpes and shingles. BIOGLAN

Vivalan
Tablets containing viloxazine hydrochloride for the symptoms of depression, especially where sedation is not required. ICI

Voltarol Emulgel
A gel containing diclofenac diethylammonium to relieve pain and inflammation in trauma of the tendons, ligaments, muscles and joints for example due to sprain, strains and bruises and also localised forms of soft tissue rheumatism. GEIGY

Voltarol, Voltarol Retard, Voltarol Dispersable
Tablets containing diclofenac used to treat arthritis, frozen shoulder, tendinitis, tenosynovitis, bursitis, sprain, strains and dislocations, gout, relief of pain in fractures, and in control of pain and inflammation in orthopaedic, dental and other minor surgery. Also available as suppositories and ampoules for injection. GEIGY

Waxsol
Liquid containing docusate sodium (a wax softener) for softening ear wax. NORGINE

Welldorm
Tablets containing chloral hydrate for the short-term treatment of insomnia. SMITH & NEPHEW

Xylocaine Ointment 5%
A topical anaesthetic ointment containing lignocaine for temporary

relief of pain associated with minor burns and abrasions of the skin, for example, herpes zoster and labialis, pruritus, sore nipples, insect bites. ASTRA

xylometazoline nasal drops
Drops to clear a blocked nose.

Xyloproct Ointment
Ointment containing lidocaine (a local anesthetic) and hydrocortisone acetate (a corticosteroid) for the relief of symptoms such as anal and vulval itching, pain and inflammation associated with piles, and other anal conditions. Suppositories available which also contain zinc oxide and aluminium acetate. ASTRA

Zantac Syrup/Tablets
Tablets or syrup containing ranitidine for ulcers, indigestion, oesophagitis, and to prevent ulcers in arthritis treatment, for example. GLAXO

Zarontin
Elixir or capsules containing ethosuximide for the treatment of epilepsy particularly petit mal epilepsy. PARKE DAVIS

Zestosretic
Tablets containing lisinopril (an antihypertensive drug) and hydrochlorothiazide (a diuretic) for the treatment of high blood pressure in patients who have been stabilised on the individual drugs given in the same proportions, but previously they were given as separate tablets. ICI

Zestril
Tablets containing lisinopril (an antihypertensive drug) for the treatment of high blood pressure and also congestive heart failure. ICI

Zimovane
Tablets containing zopiclone (a non-benzodiazepine hypnotic agent) used in the short treatment of insomnia in situations where the insomnia is debilitating or is causing severe distress for the patient. RHONE-POULENC RORER

Zinamide
Tablets containing pyrazinamide, an antituberculosis agent for use with other such agents. MERCK SHARP & DOHME LTD

Zinnat Suspension or Tablets
Suspension or tablets containing cefuroxime (an antibiotic). Uses include the treatment of respiratory tract infections, genito-urinary

tract infections, skin and soft tissue infections and gonorrhoea. GLAXO

Zineryt
An anti-inflammatory and anti-bacterial topical treatment for acne containing zinc acetate and erythromycin. BROCADES

Zocor
Tablets containing simvastatin for high cholesterol. MERCK SHARP & DOHME LTD

Zofran tablets
Tablets containing ondansetron (an anti-emetic) for nausea and vomiting as a result of medical treatments such as chemotherapy, for example. GLAXO

Zovirax Cream
Cream containing acyclovir (an anti-viral drug) for the treatment of herpes simplex virus infections of the skin. WELLCOME

Zovirax Shingles Treatment Pack
Tablets containing acyclovir (an anti-viral drug) for the treatment of herpes zoster (shingles) infections. WELLCOME

Zovirax Tablets or Suspension
Tablets and suspension containing acyclovir for the treatment of herpes simplex virus infections of the skin and mucous membranes including initial and recurrent genital herpes. WELLCOME

Zumenon
Tablets containing oestradiol for the treatment of symptoms of oestrogen deficiency as a result of natural menopause or oophorectomy (surgical removal of the functioning ovaries which causes an 'unnatural' menopause). Duphar

Zyloric
Tablets containing allopurinol uses include gout. WELLCOME

GLOSSARY

Analgesic Painkiller – aspirin, paracetamol, ibuprofen.

Antibiotic A 'naturally' produced substance which destroys or inhibits the growth of germs within the body.

Anticholinergic A chemical that prevents the passage of impulses down 'reflex' nerve pathways in the body and so can relieve symptoms or produce a beneficial effect. The substance hyoscine can do this. It is used in medicines which prevent the bowel cramps associated with irritable bowel syndrome.

Anti-inflammatory A medicine which reduces the swelling, redness, pain and overheating in inflamed tissues of the body. These can be caused by the damage of an accident, an infection or an allergy. A common example is aspirin, which can be given to remove such an inflammation – and the associated pain – in an arthritic joint, for example.

Antipyretic A medicine which helps to bring down the body's temperature, which rises when an infection is present. Such a rise in temperature can, in itself, cause feelings of illness. Paracetamol and aspirin are antipyretics.

Antispasmodic A medicine taken to relieve spasm in muscles (also see anticholinergic).

Ethical drugs A term used to describe all drugs which, irrespective of their legal category, are promoted to and prescribed by doctors. Ethical drugs are not promoted to the public.

Generic drugs The generic (or non-proprietary) name of a medicine is the name of the active ingredient. Several different brands may contain the same active ingredient. Doctors these days are encouraged to prescribe generic medicines because they are usually cheaper than other brands and can be equally effective.

Keratolytic An application which dissolves the top, hard, non-living layers of the skin, which are made up of keratin. This can make it easier for effective medicines to penetrate into the deeper, living layers of the skin.

Legal categories There are three legal categories covering medicines.

GSL General Sales List
P Pharmacy only
POM Prescription only medicine

But all three categories may be prescribed under the NHS (unless otherwise blacklisted)

An NHS prescription A prescription written by a doctor, normally on an official 'FP10' ('GP10' in Scotland) form (if the doctor is a GP), which the pharmacist will dispense to the patient. The drug(s) named on the NHS prescription will be deemed necessary by the doctor, and may be one of the three legal categories. For those patients who are not exempt, the current NHS prescription charge is £4.25 per item dispensed.

Prostaglandin A naturally occurring chemical, widely spread throughout the body and involved in regulating blood pressure or body temperature; the way in which the blood clots; the acid secretion within the stomach; and in the control of inflammation – to mention only a few.

Vasoconstrictor A substance which constricts the tiny arteries – the arterioles – and can prevent or treat congestion as a result.

Vasodilator A medicine that widens blood vessels.

USEFUL ORGANISATIONS

Arthritis Care, 18 Stephenson Way, London, NW1 2HD. Telephone: 071 916 1500.

Association of the British Pharmaceutical Industry (ABPI), 12 Whitehall, London SW1A 2DY.

British Diabetic Association (BDA), 10 Queen Anne Street, London, W1M 0BD. Telephone: 071 323 1531.

British Epilepsy Association, Anstey House, 40 Hanover Square, Leeds, LS3 1BE. Telephone: 0532 439393.

British Heart Foundation, 14 Fitzhardinge Street, London, W1H 4DH. Telephone: 071 935 0185.

Endometriosis Society, 35 Belgrave Square, London, SW1X 8QB. Telephone: 071 235 4137.

MASTA, Medical Advisory Services for Travellers Abroad, Keppel Street, London, WC1E 7HT. Telephone: 071 631 4408.

National Eczema Society, 4 Tavistock Place, London, WC1H 9RA. Telephone: 071 388 4097.

Parkinson's Disease Society of the United Kingdom, 22 Upper Woburn Place, London, WC1H ORA. Telephone: 071 383 3513.

Psoriasis Association, 7 Milton Street, Northampton, NN2 7UG. Telephone 0604 711129.

The British Migraine Association, 178a High Road, Byfleet, Weybridge, Surrey, KT14 7ED. Telephone: 0932 352468.

The Stroke Association, CHSA House, 123–127 Whitecross Street, London, EC1Y 8JJ. Telephone: 071 387 3012.

The Hospital for Tropical Diseases Travel Clinic, Queens House, 180–182 Tottenham Court Road, London W1P 9LE. Telephone: 071 637 9899.

The Migraine Trust, 45 Gt. Ormond Street, London, WC1N 3HD. Telephone: 071 278 2676.